NURSING:
A BIBLIOGRAPHY WITH INDEXES

NURSING:
A BIBLIOGRAPHY WITH INDEXES

NANCY R. VENNETI (EDITOR)

Nova Science Publishers, Inc.
New York

Senior Editors: Susan Boriotti and Donna Dennis
Coordinating Editor: Tatiana Shohov
Office Manager: Annette Hellinger
Graphics: Wanda Serrano
Editorial Production: Jennifer Vogt, Matthew Kozlowski, Jonathan Rose
and Maya Columbus
Circulation: Ave Maria Gonzalez, Indah Becker, Raymond Davis,
Vladimir Klestov and Jonathan Roque
Communications and Acquisitions: Serge P. Shohov
Marketing: Cathy DeGregory

Library of Congress Cataloging-in-Publication Data
Available Upon Request

ISBN 1-59033-312-8.

Copyright © 2002 by Nova Science Publishers, Inc.
400 Oser Ave, Suite 1600
Hauppauge, New York 11743
Tele. 631-231-7269   Fax 631-231-8175
e-mail: Novascience@earthlink.net
Web Site: http://www.novapubishers.com

Printed in the United States of America

Contents

PREFACE

A severe shortage of nurses is being experienced nationally and globally. Part of the problem is connected to the relentless practices of the so-called healthcare organizations including medical groups and hospitals which often insist on 16 hour days with little or no notice. Another part of the problem rests with doctors who continue to offput more and more medical care decisions to nurses by patient neglect. Finally the nurses themselves feel exploited and underpaid compared to the workloads and responsibilities being heaped on them. This bibliography presents carefully selected review citations to the nursing literature which are then indexed by subject, title and author.

BIBLIOGRAPHY–BOOKS

A Financial guide for nurses: investing in
yourself and others / Dorothy J. del Bueno,
editor.
Edition Information: 1st ed.
Published/Created: Boston: Blackwell
Scientific Publications, c1981.
Related Authors: Del Bueno, Dorothy J.
Description: x, 224 p.; 24 cm. ISBN:
0865420076
Notes: Bibliography: p. 211-212.
Subjects: Nursing--Vocational guidance.
Nurses--Finance, Personal.
LC Classification: RT82 .F53
Dewey Class No.: 332.024/613 19

Alexander, Jeffrey A.
Nursing unit organization, its effect on
staff professionalism / by Jeffrey A.
Alexander.
Published/Created: Ann Arbor, Mich.:
UMI Research Press, c1982.
Description: xiii, 150 p.; 24 cm. ISBN:
0835713695
Notes: Includes index. Bibliography: p.
[145]-148.
Subjects: Nursing--Vocational guidance.
Nurses--Employment. Hospitals--Staff.
Series: Studies in nursing management; no.
4
LC Classification: RT82 .A43 1982
Dewey Class No.: 305/.9613 19

American Nurses' Association Professional
Counseling and Placement Service, Inc.
The older nurse. [Report of a project on the
older nurse]
Published/Created: New York, 1954.
Description: 40 p. illus. 23 cm.
Subjects: Nursing--Vocational guidance.
LC Classification: RT82 .A6
Dewey Class No.: 610.73069

Anastas, Lila.
Your career in nursing / Lila Anastas.
Published/Created: New York: National
League for Nursing, c1984.
Description: viii, 215 p.: ill.; 23 cm. ISBN:
0887370748 (pbk.)
Notes: "Pub. no. 41-1952." Includes
bibliographical references and index.
Subjects: Nursing--Vocational guidance.
LC Classification: RT82 .A66 1984
Dewey Class No.: 610.73/023/73 19

Bartos, Linda.
New careers for nurses / by Linda Bartos.
Published/Created: Detroit, Mich. (P.O.
Box 07158, Detroit 48207): NIMCO,
c1981.
Description: 69 p.; 28 cm.
Notes: Includes bibliographies.
Subjects: Nursing--Vocational guidance.
Nurses--Employment. Career changes.
LC Classification: RT82 .B27
Dewey Class No.: 610.73/069 19

Benner, Patricia E.
The new nurse's work entry: a troubled
sponsorship / Patricia Benner, Richard V.
Benner.

Published/Created: New York: Tiresias Press, c1979.
Related Authors: Benner, Richard V., joint author.
Description: 160 p.: ill.; 21 cm. ISBN: 0913292095
Notes: Includes index. Bibliography: p. 116-120.
Subjects: Nursing--Vocational guidance. Nurses--Employment. Nursing--Study and teaching. Professional socializaton. Nurses--Rating of. Role conflict.
LC Classification: RT82 .B72
Dewey Class No.: 610.73/023

Bentling, Sonia.
I idéernas värld: en analys av omvårdnad som vetenskap och grund för en professionell utbildning / Sonia Bentling.
Published/Created: Uppsala: Academia Ubsaliensis; Stockholm: Distributor, Almqvist & Wiksell International, 1992.
Description: 197 p.; 25 cm. ISBN: 9155429688
Notes: Summary in English. Thesis (doctoral)--Uppsala universitet, 1992. Includes bibliographical references (p. 186-197)
Subjects: Nursing--Study and teaching. Nursing--Vocational guidance. Professional education.
Series: Acta Universitatis Upsaliensis. Uppsala studies in education, 0347-1314; 45
LC Classification: RT73 .B37 1992

Berglind, Hans, 1930-
Valet mellan hem och yrke. En sociologisk analys av en valsituation med tillämpning på gifta sjuksköterskor.
Published/Created: Stockholm, Norstedt, 1968.
Description: 357 p. 25 cm.
Notes: Issued also as thesis, Stockholms universitet. Issued also in series: Stockholms kommunalförvaltning. Monografier, nr. 30. Summary in English. Bibliography: p. 353-357.

Subjects: Nursing--Vocational guidance. Nurses and nursing--Sweden.
LC Classification: RT12.S7 B44 1968b
National Bib. No.: S68-25/26

Bozell, Jeanna.
Anatomy of a job search: a nurse's guide to finding and landing the job you want / Jeanna Bozell.
Published/Created: Springhouse, Pa.: Springhouse Corp., 1999.
Projected Pub. Date: 9903
Description: p. cm. ISBN: 0874349508 (alk. paper)
Notes: Includes index.
Subjects: Nursing--Vocational guidance. Nurses--Employment. Job hunting. Job Application--nurses' instruction.
LC Classification: RT86.7 .B69 1999
Dewey Class No.: 610.73/06/9 21

Bressler, Marvin.
Career dynamics; a survey of selected aspects of the nursing profession [by] Marvin Bressler and William Kephart. A Study conducted for the Pennsylvania Nurses Association under a grant from the American Nurses Assocation.
Published/Created: Harrisburg, Pennsylvania Nurses Association, 1955, c1957.
Related Authors: Kephart, William M. joint author. Pennsylvania Nurses Association.
Description: 201 p. tables. 28 cm.
Notes: Bibliographical footnotes.
Subjects: Nursing--Vocational guidance.
LC Classification: RT82 .B73
Dewey Class No.: 610.73069

Brink-Tjebbes, J. A. van den, 1924-
De theorie van de verpleegkunde, naar haar aard en functie gedacht: verslag van een denkproces / voltrokken door J. A. Tjebbes.
Published/Created: Lochem: Tijdstroom, 1975.
Description: 85 p.; 23 cm. ISBN:

906087840X:
Notes: Includes bibliographical references.
Subjects: Nursing. Nursing--Vocational
guidance.
LC Classification: RT42 .T55
National Bib. No.: Ne75-23

Brown, Esther Lucile, 1898-
Nursing as a profession, by Esther Lucile
Brown...
Published/Created: New York, Russell
Sage foundation [c1936]
Description: 2 p. 1., 120 p. incl. tables. 21
cm.
Notes: "This monograph is one of a series
dealing with the present status of certain
established or emerging professions in the
United States."--Pref.
Subjects: Nursing--Vocational guidance.
Nurses and nursing--Study and teaching.
LC Classification: RT71 .B75
Dewey Class No.: 610.73

Burke, Shelly.
How to find your perfect job in nursing /
by Shelly Burke and Martha Whited.
Published/Created: Freeman, S.D.: Pine
Hill Press, Inc., c1997.
Related Authors: Whited, Martha.
Description: xiii, 203 p.: ill.; 23 cm. ISBN:
1575790521
Subjects: Nursing--Vocational guidance.
Nurses--Employment. Nursing. Job
Satisfaction.
LC Classification: RT82 .B797 1997
Dewey Class No.: 610.73/06/9 21

Bush, Christine H.
Personal and vocational relationships for
practical nurses.
Published/Created: Philadelphia, W. B.
Saunders Co., 1961.
Description: 107 p. 21 cm.
Subjects: Nursing--Vocational guidance.
LC Classification: RT82 .B8
Dewey Class No.: 610.73069
National Bib. No.: GB61-7174

Cardillo, Donna.
Your first year as a nurse: making the
transition from total novice to successful
professional / Donna Cardillo.
Published/Created: Roseville, Calif.: Prima
Pub., 2001.
Projected Pub. Date: 0105
Description: p. cm. ISBN: 0761533338
Notes: Includes index.
Subjects: Nursing--Vocational guidance.
Nursing--Philosophy.
Series: Your first year series VERIFIER:
please check series
Variant Series: Your first year
LC Classification: RT42 .C32 2001
Dewey Class No.: 610.73/06/9 21

Career planning for nurses / [edited by] Bette
Case.
Published/Created: Albany: Delmar
Publishers, c1997.
Related Authors: Case, Bette.
Description: xvii, 362 p.: ill.; 23 cm. ISBN:
0827371659
Notes: Includes bibliographical references
and index.
Subjects: Nursing--Vocational guidance.
Career Mobility. Nursing. Vocational
Guidance.
LC Classification: RT82 .C285 1997
Dewey Class No.: 610.73/06/9 20

Careers in focus. Nursing.
Published/Created: Chicago, IL: Ferguson
Pub., c2001.
Related Authors: J.G. Ferguson Publishing
Company.
Description: 184 p.: ill.; 24 cm. ISBN:
0894343203
Notes: Includes index.
Subjects: Nursing--Vocational guidance.
Nursing--Vocational guidance. Vocational
guidance.
LC Classification: RT82 .C288 2001
Dewey Class No.: 610.73/06/9 21 lcac

Careers in nursing, 1967; with a foreword by
Julian Snow; editor John Callaghan.

Published/Created: London, Classic
Publications [1967]
Related Authors: Callaghan, John, ed.
Description: 84, [12] p. 22 cm.
Notes: Form as insert.
Subjects: Nursing--Vocational guidance.
Nursing--Great Britain. Schools, Nursing--
directories.
LC Classification: RT82
Dewey Class No.: 610.73
National Bib. No.: B68-02310

Careers in nursing, 1969: editor John Callaghan
with a foreword by Julian Snow.
Published/Created: London, Classic
Publications [1969]
Related Authors: Callaghan, John, ed.
Description: 80 p. illus., coat of arms, map.
22 cm.
Subjects: Nursing--Vocational guidance.
Nursing--Great Britain--yearbooks.
Schools, Nursing--Great Britain--direct.
LC Classification: RT82
Dewey Class No.: 610.73/023
National Bib. No.: B69-12068

Carson, Ruth, 1903-
How we can get the nurses we need.
Edition Information: [1st ed.
Published/Created: New York, Public
Affairs Committee, 1966]
Description: 28 p. 19 cm.
Subjects: Nursing--Vocational guidance.
Variant Series: Public affairs pamphlet no.
385
LC Classification: RT82 .C3
Dewey Class No.: 610.073

Chandler, Caroline A. (Caroline Augusta),
1906-
Nursing as a career [by] Caroline A.
Chandler and Sharon H. Kempf.
Published/Created: New York, Dodd,
Mead [1970]
Related Authors: Kempf, Sharon H., joint
author.
Description: xii, 157 p. illus. 22 cm. ISBN:
039606230X

Summary: Describes nursing as a
profession, including the possible
preparatory tryouts as a volunteer, a candy
striper, a nurse's aide, and other training
leading to qualification as an R.N.
Notes: Bibliography: p. 153-154.
Subjects: Nursing--Vocational guidance.
Nursing--Vocational guidance.
LC Classification: RT82 .C48
Dewey Class No.: 610.73/023

Chayer, Mary Ella.
Nursing in modern society.
Published/Created: New York, Putnam
[1947]
Related Authors: Bixler, Genevieve
Knight, ed.
Description: xx, 288 p. 21 cm.
Notes: Ed. by Genevieve Knight Bixler.
Bibliography: p. 263-279.
Subjects: Nursing--Vocational guidance.
Series: Modern nursing
LC Classification: RT71 .C53
Dewey Class No.: 610.73069

Chenevert, Melodie, 1941-
Mosby's tour guide to nursing school: a
student's road survival kit / Melodie
Chenevert.
Edition Information: 3rd ed.
Published/Created: St. Louis: Mosby Year
Book, c1995.
Related Authors: Mosby-Year Book.
National Student Nurses' Association
(U.S.)
Related Titles: Tour guide to nursing
school.
Description: xv, 216 p.: ill.; 24 cm. ISBN:
0815115393
Notes: "In collaboration with NSNA,
National Student Nurses' Association"--P.
[i]. Includes bibliographical references (p.
173-175) and index.
Subjects: Nursing students. Nursing
schools. Nursing--Vocational guidance.
Success. Schools, Nursing--popular works.
Education, Nursing--popular works.
LC Classification: RT73 .C49 1995

Dewey Class No.: 610.73/071/1 20

Chenevert, Melodie, 1941-
Mosby's tour guide to nursing school: a
student's road survival kit / Melodie
Chenevert.
Published/Created: St. Louis: Mosby,
1987.
Related Authors: C.V. Mosby Company.
Related Titles: Tour guide to nursing
school.
Description: xiv, 184 p.: ill.; 24 cm. ISBN:
0801613183 (pbk.)
Subjects: Nursing students. Nursing
schools. Nursing--Vocational guidance.
Success. Education, Nursing--popular
works. Schools, Nursing--popular works.
LC Classification: RT73 .C49 1987
Dewey Class No.: 610.73/0711 19

Clark, Marguerite (Sheridan), 1900-
The nurse everyone needs. In cooperation
with the National Association for Practical
Nurse Education and Service, inc.
Edition Information: [1st ed.
Published/Created: New York, Public
Affairs Committee, 1963]
Description: 28 p. illus. 18 cm.
Subjects: Nursing--Vocational guidance.
Practical nursing.
Variant Series: Public affairs pamphlet no.
338
LC Classification: RT82 .C55

Colwell, Max.
Careers in nursing.
Published/Created: [Melbourne]
Macmillan of Australia, 1968.
Description: 53 p. 18 cm.
Subjects: Nursing--Vocational guidance.
Variant Series: Career books
LC Classification: RT82 .C57
Dewey Class No.: 610.73/023
National Bib. No.: Aus68-2267

Davis, Fred, 1925- ed.
The nursing profession: five sociological
essays.

Published/Created: New York, Wiley
[1966]
Description: xii, 203 p. illus. 24 cm.
Contents: Nursing leadership and policy:
some cross-national comparison, by W. A.
Glaser.--The structure and ideology of
American nursing: an interpretation, by A.
Strauss.--The organizational context of
nursing practice, by H. O. Mauksch.--
Problems and issues in collegiate nursing
education, by F. Davis, V. L. Olesen, and
E. W. Whittaker.--Nursing and patient
care, by E. L. Brown.
Notes: Includes bibliographies.
Subjects: Nursing--Vocational guidance.
LC Classification: RT63 .D35
Dewey Class No.: 610.73

Deming, Dorothy, 1893-
Careers for nurses.
Edition Information: 2d ed.
Published/Created: New York, McGraw-
Hill, 1952.
Description: 351 p. 24 cm.
Subjects: Nursing--Vocational guidance.
Variant Series: McGraw-Hill series in
nursing
LC Classification: RT82 .D4 1952
Dewey Class No.: 610.69
National Bib. No.: GB52-8588

Deming, Dorothy, 1893-
Careers for nurses.
Edition Information: 1st ed.
Published/Created: New York, McGraw-
Hill, 1947.
Description: xiv, 358 p. illus. 24 cm.
Subjects: Nursing--Vocational guidance.
Variant Series: McGraw-Hill series in
nursing
LC Classification: RT82 .D4 1947
Dewey Class No.: 610.69

Developing your career in nursing / edited by
Desmond F.S. Cormack.
Edition Information: 1st ed.
Published/Created: London; New York:
Chapman and Hall, 1990.

Related Authors: Cormack, Desmond.
Description: xi, 301 p.: ill.; 24 cm. ISBN:
0412321300
Notes: Includes bibliographical references
and index.
Subjects: Nursing--Great Britain--
Vocational guidance. Nursing--Vocational
guidance. Career development--Great
Britain. Career development. Career
Choice. Clinical Competence. Education,
Nursing, Continuing. Nursing.
LC Classification: RT82 .D47 1990
Dewey Class No.: 610.73/06/9 20

DeYoung, Lillian.
The foundations of nursing as conceived,
learned, and practiced in professional
nursing.
Published/Created: Saint Louis, C. V.
Mosby Co., 1966.
Description: xii, 279 p. illus. 25 cm.
Notes: Includes bibliographies.
Subjects: Nursing--Vocational guidance.
LC Classification: RT82 .D48
Dewey Class No.: 610.73023

Dietz, Lena Dixon, 1890-
History and modern nursing [by] Lena
Dixon Dietz [and] Aurelia R. Lehozky.
Edition Information: 2d ed.
Published/Created: Philadelphia, F.A.
Davis Co. [1967]
Related Authors: Lehozky, Aurelia R.,
joint author.
Description: 381 p. illus. 27 cm.
Notes: Includes bibliographies.
Subjects: Nursing--History. Nursing--
Vocational guidance.
LC Classification: RT31 .D5 1967
Dewey Class No.: 610.73/09

Dietz, Lena Dixon, 1890-
History and modern nursing.
Published/Created: Philadelphia, F.A.
Davis [1963]
Description: 365 p. illus. 27 cm.
Notes: Includes bibliography.
Subjects: Nursing--History. Nursing--

Vocational guidance.
LC Classification: RT31 .D5
Dewey Class No.: 610.7309

Dodge, Bertha Sanford, 1902-
The story of nursing / by Bertha S. Dodge;
illustrated by Barbara Corrigan.
Edition Information: New ed.
Published/Created: Boston: Little, Brown,
[1965]
Description: x, 244 p.: ill.; 22 cm.
Notes: Includes bibliographical references
(p. [233]-238) and index.
Subjects: Nursing--History. Nursing--
Vocational guidance.
LC Classification: RT31 .D62 1965
Dewey Class No.: 610.7309

Doheny, Margaret O'Bryan, 1948-
The discipline of nursing: an introduction /
Margaret O'Bryan Doheny, Christina
Benson Cook, Mary Constance Stopper.
Edition Information: 4th ed.
Published/Created: Stamford, Conn.:
Appleton & Lange, c1997.
Related Authors: Cook, Christina Benson.
Stopper, Mary Constance, 1944-
Description: vi, 300 p.: ill.; 23 cm. ISBN:
0838517161 (pbk.: alk. paper)
Notes: Includes bibliographical references
and index.
Subjects: Nursing--Vocational guidance.
Nursing. Nursing.
LC Classification: RT82 .D63 1997
Dewey Class No.: 610.73/06/9 20

Doheny, Margaret O'Bryan, 1948-
The discipline of nursing: an introduction /
Margaret O'Bryan Doheny, Christina
Benson Cook, Mary Constance Stopper.
Edition Information: 3rd ed.
Published/Created: Norwalk, Conn.:
Appleton & Lange, c1992.
Related Authors: Cook, Christina Benson.
Stopper, Mary Constance, 1944-
Description: vi, 258 p.: ill.; 23 cm. ISBN:
0838517145
Notes: Includes bibliographical references

and index.
Subjects: Nursing--Vocational guidance.
Nursing. Nursing.
LC Classification: RT82 .D63 1992
Dewey Class No.: 610.73/069 20

Doheny, Margaret O'Bryan, 1948-
The discipline of nursing: an introduction /
Margaret O'Bryan Doheny, Christina
Benson Cook, Mary Constance Stopper.
Edition Information: 2nd ed.
Published/Created: East Norwalk, Conn.:
Appleton & Lange, c1987.
Related Authors: Cook, Christina Benson.
Stopper, Mary Constance, 1944-
Description: xi, 258 p.: ill.; 23 cm. ISBN:
0838517153 (pbk.)
Notes: Includes bibliographies and index.
Subjects: Nursing--Vocational guidance.
Nursing. Nursing.
LC Classification: RT82 .D63 1987
Dewey Class No.: 610.73/069 19

Doheny, Margaret O'Bryan, 1948-
The discipline of nursing: an introduction /
Margaret O'Bryan Doheny, Christina
Benson Cook, Mary Constance Stopper.
Published/Created: Bowie, Md.: R.J. Brady
Co., c1982.
Related Authors: Cook, Christina Benson.
Stopper, Mary Constance, 1944-
Description: xi, 208 p.: ill.; 23 cm. ISBN:
0893030589:
Notes: Includes bibliographies and index.
Subjects: Nursing. Nursing--Vocational
guidance.
LC Classification: RT82 .D63 1982
Dewey Class No.: 610.73/069 19

Downs, Florence S.
New careers in nursing / Florence Downs
and Dorothy Brooten.
Published/Created: New York: Arco Pub.,
c1983.
Related Authors: Brooten, Dorothy A.
Description: ix, 180 p.: ill.; 26 cm. ISBN:
0668052554: 0668052600 (pbk.):
Notes: Includes bibliographical references

and index.
Subjects: Nursing--Vocational guidance.
Specialties, Nursing.
LC Classification: RT82 .D68 1983
Dewey Class No.: 610.73/06/9 19

Ducas, Dorothy, 1904-
Modern nursing.
Published/Created: New York, H.Z.
Walck, 1962.
Description: 111 p. illus. 22 cm.
Subjects: Nursing--Vocational guidance.
Variant Series: Careers for tomorrow
LC Classification: RT82 .D8
Dewey Class No.: 610.73069

Eagles, Zardoya E.
The nurses' career guide: discovering new
horizons in health care / Zardoya E.
Eagles.
Published/Created: San Luis Obispo, CA:
Sovreignty Press, c1997.
Description: xii, 240 p.: ill.; 23 cm. ISBN:
0965602583
Notes: Includes bibliographical references
(p. 171-175) and index.
Subjects: Nursing--Vocational guidance.
LC Classification: RT82 .E24 1997
Dewey Class No.: 610.73/06/9 21

EMNID GmbH & Co.
Die gesellschaftliche Einschätzung von
Krankenpflegeberufen in der
Bundesrepublik Deutschland. 1.
Ergebnisse von Umfragen bei jungen
Mädchen und in der Bevölkerung. 2.
Ergebnisse von Umfragen bei jungen
Männern und in der Bevölkerung.
(Durchgeführt vom EMNID-Institut GmbH
& Co., Bielefeld.)
Published/Created: [Bochum]
Studienstiftung der Verwaltungsleiter
Deutscher Krankenanstalten e.V. (1969).
Description: 357 p. illus. 21 cm.
Subjects: Nursing--Germany (East)--
Statistics. Nursing--Vocational guidance.
Nursing--Germany, West.
Series: [Fachvereinigung der

Verwaltungsleiter Deutscher
Krankenanstalten. Schriftenreihe] Bd. 22
LC Classification: RT12.G3 E4
National Bib. No.: GDNB69-B20-247

Ferreira-Santos, Célia Almeida.
A enfermagem como profissão (estudo
num hospital-escola).
Published/Created: São Paulo, Livraria
Pioneira Editôra [1973]
Description: 176 p. 21cm.
Notes: Bibliography: p. 171-176.
Subjects: Nursing--Vocational guidance.
Variant Series: Biblioteca Pioneira de
ciências sociais: sociologia
LC Classification: RT82 .F4

Frederickson, Keville.
Opportunities in nursing / Keville
Frederickson.
Published/Created: Louisville, Ky.:
Vocational Guidance Manuals, c1977.
Description: 148 p.: ill.; 20 cm. ISBN:
0890222320. 0890222339
Summary: Surveys the scope and history of
nursing and discusses the education and
training necessary to enter the field, types
and places of employment, how to obtain a
job, and professional organizations.
Notes: Includes index.
Subjects: Nursing--Vocational guidance.
Nursing--Vocational guidance. Vocational
guidance.
LC Classification: RT82 .F65
Dewey Class No.: 610.73/023

Gillam, Robert.
Schoolgirls' interest in nursing as a career.
Research assistant: Anthony Cable.
Published/Created: [Kensington, Sydney]
University of New South Wales, School of
Hospital Administration, 1968.
Related Authors: Cable, Anthony.
Description: 38 l. tables. 26 cm.
Subjects: Nursing--Vocational guidance.
Series: Australian studies in health service
administration no. 3
LC Classification: RA421 .A94 no. 3

Dewey Class No.: 610.73/023
National Bib. No.: Aus68-3622rev

Hafner, Betty.
The nurse's guide to starting a small
business / by Betty Hafner.
Published/Created: Babylon, N.Y.: Pilot
Books, c1992.
Description: 48 p.; 22 cm. ISBN:
0875761631:
Notes: Includes bibliographical references
(p. 38-39).
Subjects: Nursing--Vocational guidance.
Nursing consultants--Vocational guidance.
Career changes. Nursing--Practice. New
business enterprises. Career Mobility.
Entrepreneurship. Nursing.
LC Classification: RT82 .H34 1992
Dewey Class No.: 362.1/73/0681 20

Hafner, Betty.
Where do I go from here?: exploring your
career alternatives within and beyond
clinical nursing / by Betty Hafner.
Published/Created: Philadelphia:
Lippincott, c2002.
Projected Pub. Date: 0108
Description: p.; cm. ISBN: 0781734924
(alk. paper)
Notes: Includes bibliographical references
and index.
Subjects: Nursing--Vocational guidance.
Nurses--Employment. Job hunting.
Nursing--United States. Career Mobility--
United States.
LC Classification: RT86.7 .H345 2002
Dewey Class No.: 610.73/06/9 21

Hamilton, Persis Mary.
Realities of contemporary nursing / Persis
Mary Hamilton.
Edition Information: 2nd ed.
Published/Created: Menlo Park, CA:
Addison-Wesley Nursing, c1996.
Description: xi, 467 p.: ill.; 24 cm. ISBN:
0805320202
Notes: Includes bibliographical references
and index.

Subjects: Nursing--Vocational guidance.
Nursing--Practice. Nursing. Philosophy,
Nursing.
LC Classification: RT82 .H35 1996
Dewey Class No.: 610.73 20

Hanton, E. Michael.
The new nurse, by E. Michael Hanton.
Edition Information: [1st ed.
Published/Created: Bangor, Me., L. H.
Thompson, 1973]
Description: vi, 122 p. 23 cm.
Subjects: Nursing--Vocational guidance.
LC Classification: RT82 .H36
Dewey Class No.: 610.73/069

Harrington, Nicki.
LPN to RN transitions / Nicki Harrington,
Nancy E. Smith, Wanda E. Spratt.
Published/Created: Philadelphia:
Lippincott, c1996.
Related Authors: Smith, Nancy E. (Nancy
Ellen), 1949- Spratt, Wanda E.
Description: xvii, 398 p.: ill.; 23 cm. ISBN:
0397550650
Notes: Includes bibliographical references
and index.
Subjects: Nursing--Vocational guidance.
Practical nurses. Nursing--examination
questions. Nursing, Practical. Nurses--
psychology. Career Mobility.
LC Classification: RT82 .H37 1996
Dewey Class No.: 610.73/06/9 20

Henderson, Frances C.
Managing your career in nursing / Frances
C. Henderson, Barbara O. McGettigan.
Edition Information: 2nd ed.
Published/Created: New York: National
League for Nursing Press, c1994.
Related Authors: McGettigan, Barbara O.
Description: ix, 358 p.: ill.; 24 cm. ISBN:
0887376290
Notes: "Pub. No. 14-2640." Includes
bibliographical references and index.
Subjects: Nursing--Vocational guidance.
LC Classification: RT82 .H46 1994

Dewey Class No.: 610.73/06/9 20

Henderson, Frances C.
Managing your career in nursing / Frances
C. Henderson, Barbara O. McGettigan.
Published/Created: Reading, Mass.:
Addison-Wesley, c1986.
Related Authors: McGettigan, Barbara O.
Description: xii, 276 p.: ill.; 24 cm. ISBN:
0201129582 (pbk.)
Notes: Includes index. Bibliography: p.
259-267.
Subjects: Nursing--Vocational guidance.
Career Mobility. Nursing.
LC Classification: RT82 .H46 1986
Dewey Class No.: 610.73/023 19

Heron, Jackie.
Exploring careers in nursing / by Jackie
Heron.
Edition Information: 1st ed.
Published/Created: New York: Rosen Pub.
Group, 1986.
Description: v, 131 p.: ill.; 22 cm. ISBN:
0823906892:
Notes: Includes index.
Subjects: Nursing--Vocational guidance.
Career Choice. Nursing.
LC Classification: RT82 .H47 1986
Dewey Class No.: 610.73/023 19

Hoffman, Vicki Reynolds.
New directions for the professional nurse:
exploring your career options and
discovering great escapes / Vicki Reynolds
Hoffman.
Published/Created: New York: Arco Pub.,
c1984.
Description: xiv, 225 p.: ill.; 25 cm. ISBN:
0668055642: 0668052996 (pbk.):
Notes: Includes index. Bibliography: p.
223.
Subjects: Nursing--Vocational guidance.
Nurses--Attitudes. Nursing. Career
mobility. Job satisfaction.
LC Classification: RT82 .H63 1984
Dewey Class No.: 610.73/069 19

Joel, Lucille A.
The nursing experience: trends, challenges, and transitions / Lucille A. Joel, Lucie Young Kelly.
Edition Information: 4th ed.
Published/Created: New York: McGraw-Hill, c2002.
Related Authors: Kelly, Lucie Young.
Description: xvii, 767 p.: ill.; 23 cm. ISBN: 0071363157 (pbk.: alk. paper)
Notes: Includes bibliographical references (p. 621-640) and index.
Subjects: Nursing--Vocational guidance. Nursing. Nursing.
LC Classification: RT82 .K43 2002
Dewey Class No.: 610.73 21

Katz, Janet R., 1953-
Majoring in nursing: from prerequisites to post graduate study and beyond / Janet R. Katz.
Edition Information: 1st ed.
Published/Created: New York: Farrar, Straus and Giroux, 1999.
Description: 130 p.; 24 cm. ISBN: 0374525676 (alk. paper)
Subjects: Nursing--Vocational guidance.
LC Classification: RT82 .K35 1999
Dewey Class No.: 610.73/06/09 21

Kay, Eleanor.
Nurses and what they do.
Published/Created: New York, F. Watts [1968]
Description: 123 p. 22 cm.
Summary: Describes all types of nursing inside and outside the hospital, the education needed to become a nurse, various training programs, and career opportunities in nursing now and in the future.
Subjects: Nursing--Vocational guidance. Nursing--Vocational guidance.
LC Classification: RT82 .K38
Dewey Class No.: 610.73

Kearney, Rose.
Advancing your career: concepts of professional nursing / Rose Kearney.
Edition Information: 2nd ed.
Published/Created: Philadelphia: F.A. Davis Co., c2001.
Description: xxi, 498 p.: ill.; 26 cm. ISBN: 0803608071 (pbk.)
Notes: Includes bibliographical references and index.
Subjects: Nursing--Vocational guidance. Career development. Nursing--Vocational guidance--United States. Nursing--Philosophy.
LC Classification: RT82 .N85 2001
Dewey Class No.: 610.73/06/9 21

Kearney, Rose.
Advancing your career: concepts of professional nursing / Rose Kearney Nunnery.
Published/Created: Philadelphia: Davis, c1997.
Description: xxix, 424 p.: ill. (some col.); 26 cm. ISBN: 0803602359
Notes: Includes bibliographical references and index.
Subjects: Nursing--Vocational guidance. Career development. Nursing--Vocational guidance--United States. Nursing--Philosophy. Nursing. Career Mobility.
LC Classification: RT82 .N85 1997
Dewey Class No.: 610.73/06/9 21

Kelly, Cordelia W.
Dimensions of professional nursing.
Edition Information: 2d ed.
Published/Created: New York, Macmillan [1968]
Description: xiii, 494 p. 25 cm.
Notes: Includes bibliographies.
Subjects: Nursing--Vocational guidance.
LC Classification: RT82 .K4 1968
Dewey Class No.: 610.73/0692

Kelly, Cordelia W.
Dimensions of professional nursing.
Published/Created: New York, Macmillan [1962]
Description: 485 p. illus. 29 cm.

Notes: Includes bibliography.
Subjects: Nursing--Vocational guidance.
LC Classification: RT82 .K4
Dewey Class No.: 610.73069

Kelly, Lucie Young.
The nursing experience: trends, challenges, and transitions / Lucie Young Kelly; consulting editor, Madeline Renee Turkeltaub.
Published/Created: New York: Macmillan, c1987.
Related Authors: Turkeltaub, Madeline Renee.
Description: xv, 576 p.: ill.; 24 cm. ISBN: 0023635002 (pbk.)
Notes: Includes index. Bibliography: p. 514-524.
Subjects: Nursing--Vocational guidance. Nursing. Nursing. Nursing--trends.
LC Classification: RT82 .K43 1987
Dewey Class No.: 610.73 19

Kelly, Lucie Young.
The nursing experience: trends, challenges, and transitions / Lucie Young Kelly; contribution author, Sally Solomon Cohen.
Edition Information: 2nd ed.
Published/Created: New York: McGraw-Hill, c1992.
Related Authors: Cohen, Sally Solomon.
Description: xv, 637 p.: ill.; 24 cm. ISBN: 0071053905
Notes: Includes bibliographical references and index.
Subjects: Nursing--Vocational guidance. Nursing. Nursing--trends.
LC Classification: RT82 .K43 1992
Dewey Class No.: 610.73 20

Kelly, Lucie Young.
The nursing experience: trends, challenges, and transitions / Lucie Young Kelly, Lucille A. Joel.
Edition Information: 3rd ed.
Published/Created: New York: McGraw-Hill, Health Professions Division, c1996.
Related Authors: Joel, Lucille A.

Description: xvi, 763 p.: ill.; 24 cm. ISBN: 0071054839
Notes: "Bibliography": p. [617]-638. Includes bibliographical references and index.
Subjects: Nursing--Vocational guidance. Nursing. Nursing.
LC Classification: RT82 .K43 1996
Dewey Class No.: 610.73 20

Keys to nursing success / Janet R. Katz ... [et al.].
Published/Created: Upper Saddle River, N.J.: Prentice Hall, c2001.
Projected Pub. Date: 0101
Related Authors: Katz, Janet R., 1953-
Description: p.; cm. ISBN: 0130195758
Notes: Includes bibliographical references and index.
Subjects: Nursing. Nursing--Study and teaching. Nursing--Vocational guidance. Test-taking skills. Nursing. Career Choice. Education, Nursing.
LC Classification: RT71 .K49 2001
Dewey Class No.: 610.73 21

Krankendienst der Zukunft: Job oder menschl. Einsatz? / hrsg. von Hans Kramer; mit Beitr. Von Franz Josef Illhardt ... [et al.].
Edition Information: 1. Aufl.
Published/Created: Düsseldorf: Patmos-Verlag, 1974.
Related Authors: Kramer, Hans, 1936-
Description: 175 p.; 21 cm. ISBN: 3491775612:
Notes: Includes bibliographies.
Subjects: Nursing--Study and teaching--Germany. Nursing--Vocational guidance. Health care teams.
Variant Series: Patmos Paperback
LC Classification: RT12.G3 K7

Kriegel, Julia.
The head nurse; thoughts and decisions.
Published/Created: New York, Macmillan [c1968]
Description: x, 197 p. illus. 21 cm.
Notes: Bibliography: p. 189-[190]

Subjects: Nursing services--
Administration. Nursing--Vocational
guidance.
LC Classification: RT82 .K7
Dewey Class No.: 610.73

Lewis, Edith Patton.
Nurse; careers within a career in
professional nursing.
Published/Created: New York, Macmillan,
1962.
Description: x, 178 p.
Subjects: Nursing--Vocational guidance.
Variant Series: Macmillan career book
LC Classification: RT82 .L39
Dewey Class No.: 610.73069

Lewis, Edith Patton.
Opportunities in nursing.
Published/Created: New York, Vocational
Guidance Manuals [1952]
Description: 128 p. 20 cm.
Subjects: Nursing--Vocational guidance.
Variant Series: Vocational guidance
manuals
LC Classification: RT82 .L4
Dewey Class No.: 610.73069

Lotito, Mary Sue.
Advance, the nurse's guide to success in
today's job market / Mary Sue Lotito,
Joyce Kostenbauer.
Edition Information: 1st ed.
Published/Created: Boston: Little, Brown,
c1981.
Related Authors: Kostenbauer, Joyce.
Description: xii, 292 p.; 24 cm. ISBN:
0316533521 (pbk.)
Notes: Includes index. Bibliography: p.
[283]
Subjects: Nursing--Vocational guidance.
Job hunting. Nursing--Vocational
guidance--United States.
LC Classification: RT82 .L6
Dewey Class No.: 610.73/023 19

Marsh, David C. (David Charles)
Focus on nurse recruitment; a snapshot

from the provinces [by] David C. Marsh
[and] Arthur J. Willcocks.
Published/Created: London, New York,
Published for the Nuffield Provincial
Hospitals Trust by Oxford University
Press, 1965.
Related Authors: Willcocks, Arthur John,
joint author. Nuffield Provincial Hospitals
Trust.
Description: vi, 50 p. 22 cm.
Notes: Bibliographical footnotes.
Subjects: Nursing--Vocational guidance.
LC Classification: RT82 .M32
National Bib. No.: GB65-12280

Maxwell, Rachel Maureen, 1918-
Your career in nursing; the caring
profession, by R. Maureen Maxwell.
Published/Created: Nashville, Tenn.,
Southern Pub. Association [1971]
Description: 64 p. illus. 22 cm. ISBN:
0812700430
Summary: Outlines the various job
opportunities and necessary training for a
career in the nursing field.
Subjects: Nursing--Vocational guidance.
Nursing--Vocational guidance.
LC Classification: RT82 .M36
Dewey Class No.: 610.73/069

McKenna, Frances M.
Thresholds to professional nursing
practice.
Edition Information: 2d ed.
Published/Created: Philadelphia, Saunders,
1960.
Description: 428 p. illus. 22 cm.
Subjects: Nursing--Vocational guidance.
LC Classification: RT82 .M25 1960
Dewey Class No.: 610.73069
National Bib. No.: GB60-9650

McKenna, Frances M.
Thresholds to professional nursing
practice.
Published/Created: Philadelphia, Saunders,
1955.
Description: 374 p. ill. 21 cm.

Notes: Includes bibliography.
Subjects: Nursing--Vocational guidance.
LC Classification: RT82 .M25
Dewey Class No.: 610.73069
National Bib. No.: GB55-6202

Merker, Laura R.
The clinical career ladder: planning and
implementation / Laura R. Merker,
Kathleen A. Mariak, Dana W. Dwinnells.
Published/Created: New York: Springer
Pub. Co., c1985.
Related Authors: Mariak, Kathleen A.
Dwinnells, Dana W.
Description: xii, 164 p.: ill.; 21 cm. ISBN:
0826146112 (pbk.)
Notes: Includes index. Bibliography: p.
127-132.
Subjects: Nursing--Vocational guidance.
Nursing services--Administration. Career
Mobility. Nurse Clinicians. Nursing
Service, Hospital--organization &
administration. Personnel Management.
LC Classification: RT82 .M39 1985
Dewey Class No.: 362.1/73/0683 19

Meyer, Genevieve Rogge.
Tenderness and technique; nursing values
in transition.
Published/Created: Los Angeles, Institute
of Industrial Relations, University of
California [1960]
Description: 160 p. illus. 24 cm.
Notes: Includes bibliography.
Subjects: Nursing--Vocational guidance.
Variant Series: Institute of Industrial
Relations, University of California, Los
Angeles. Monograph series, 6
LC Classification: RT82 .M4
Dewey Class No.: 610.73069

Morison, Luella Josephine, 1911-
Steppingstones to professional nursing;
text and workbook for student nurses [by]
Luella J. Morison.
Edition Information: 4th ed.
Published/Created: St. Louis, C. V. Mosby
Co., 1965.

Description: 462 p. illus. (part col.) 29 cm.
Notes: Includes bibliographies.
Subjects: Nursing--Vocational guidance.
Nurses and nursing--Study and teaching.
LC Classification: RT82 .M6 1965
Dewey Class No.: 610.73069
National Bib. No.: GB65-10707

National League for Nursing. Council on
Occupational Health Nursing.
Bibliography on occupational health
nursing / National League for Nursing.
Council on Occupational Health Nursing.
Published/Created: New York: The
League, 1965.
Related Titles: Occupational health
nursing: bibliography.
Description: 15 p.; 23 cm.
Notes: Cover title. Supplements the
League's Bibliographies on nursing, v.12,
Occupational health nursing.
Subjects: Industrial nursing--Bibliography.
Nursing--Vocational guidance.
LC Classification: Z6675.I5 N3

National League of Nursing Education.
Committee on Vocational Guidance.
Handbook for career counselors on the
profession of nursing.
Published/Created: New York, National
League of Nursing Education, 1948.
Description: viii, 31 p. 23 cm.
Notes: Bibliography: p. 31.
Subjects: Nursing--Vocational guidance.
LC Classification: RT71 .N328
Dewey Class No.: 610.73069

New South Wales. Division of Vocational
Guidance Services.
Nursing.
Published/Created: [Sydney, 1968]
Description: 16 p. illus. 19 cm.
Notes: Cover title.
Subjects: Nursing--Vocational guidance.
Variant Series: Vocational guidance leaflet
LC Classification: RT82 .N4
Dewey Class No.: 610.73/023

National Bib. No.: Aus69-500

Newell, Michael.
Reinventing your nursing career: a handbook for success in the age of managed care / Michael Newell, Mario Pinardo.
Published/Created: Gaithersburg, Md.: Aspen Publishers, 1998.
Related Authors: Pinardo, Mario.
Description: xiii, 253 p.: ill.; 23 cm. ISBN: 083421007X (paper)
Notes: Includes bibliographical references and index.
Subjects: Nursing--Vocational guidance. Nursing--Effect of managed care on. Economics, Nursing--United States. Nursing Services--organization & administration--United States. Managed Care Programs--organization & administration United States. Case Management.
LC Classification: RT82 .N45 1998
Dewey Class No.: 610.73/06/9 21

Nourse, Alan Edward.
So you want to be a nurse, by Alan E. Nourse with Eleanore Halliday.
Edition Information: [1st ed.]
Published/Created: New York, Harper [1961]
Description: 186 p. 22 cm.
Subjects: Nursing--Vocational guidance.
LC Classification: RT82 .N6
Dewey Class No.: 610.7369

Novak, Gail, ed.
Your career opportunities in nursing, edited by Gail Novak with the cooperation of Margaret C. Bayldon.
Published/Created: New York, Rowan and Littlefield [c1962]
Description: 64 p. illus. 25 cm.
Notes: Includes bibliography.
Subjects: Nursing--Vocational guidance.
Variant Series: Visual career guides, no. 2
LC Classification: RT82 .N65

Dewey Class No.: 610.73069

Nowak, Janie Brown.
Career planning in nursing / Janie Brown Nowak, Cecelia Gatson Grindel; contributors, Donna Sullivan Havens, Theresa M. Valiga.
Published/Created: Philadelphia: Lippincott, c1984.
Related Authors: Grindel, Cecelia Gatson.
Description: xii, 273 p.; 23 cm. ISBN: 039754474X (pbk.)
Notes: Includes bibliographies and index.
Subjects: Nurses--Employment. Résumés (Employment) Nursing--Vocational guidance. Nursing. Career choice.
LC Classification: RT86.7 .N68 1984
Dewey Class No.: 610.73/06/9 19

Nursing education: an international perspective / edited by Grace Mashaba and Hilla Brink.
Published/Created: Kenwyn: Juta, 1994.
Related Authors: Mashaba, T. G. Brink, Hilla.
Description: xx, 332 p.: ill.; 25 cm. ISBN: 0702126209
Notes: Includes bibliographical references and index.
Subjects: Nursing schools--Faculty. Nursing--Vocational guidance. Education, Nursing--methods--essays Teaching--methods--essays Faculty, Nursing--essays
LC Classification: RT73 .N776 1994
Dewey Class No.: 610.73/071/1 20

Nursing roles: evolving or recycled? / Sue Moorhead, editor; Diane Gardner Huber, chair of the board.
Published/Created: Thousand Oaks, Calif.: Sage Publications, c1997.
Related Authors: Moorhead, Sue. Huber, Diane.
Description: xviii, 213 p.: ill.; 24 cm. ISBN: 0761901493
Notes: Includes bibliographical references and indexes.
Subjects: Nursing specialties. Nurse practitioners. Nursing--Vocational

guidance.
Series: Series on nursing administration; v. 9
LC Classification: RT86.7 .N94 1997
Dewey Class No.: 610.73/069 20

Nursing today: transition and trends / [edited by] JoAnn Zerwekh, Jo Carol Claborn.
Edition Information: 3rd ed.
Published/Created: Philadelphia: Saunders, c2000.
Related Authors: Zerwekh, JoAnn Graham. Claborn, Jo Carol.
Description: xvii, 600 p.: ill.; 24 cm. ISBN: 0721686850
Notes: Includes bibliographical references and index.
Subjects: Nursing--Vocational guidance. Nursing--Social aspects. Nursing.
LC Classification: RT82 .N874 2000
Dewey Class No.: 610.73/06/9 21

Nursing today: transition and trends / [edited by] JoAnn Zerwekh, Jo Carol Claborn.
Edition Information: 2nd ed.
Published/Created: Philadelphia: Saunders, c1997.
Related Authors: Zerwekh, JoAnn Graham. Claborn, Jo Carol.
Description: xv, 535 p.: ill.; 24 cm. ISBN: 0721668992
Notes: Includes bibliographical references and index.
Subjects: Nursing--Vocational guidance. Nursing--Social aspects. Nursing.
LC Classification: RT82 .N874 1997
Dewey Class No.: 610.73/06/9 20

Nursing today: transition and trends / [edited by] JoAnn Zerwekh, Jo Carol Claborn.
Published/Created: Philadelphia: W.B. Saunders, c1994.
Related Authors: Zerwekh, JoAnn Graham. Claborn, Jo Carol.
Description: xiv, 450 p.: ill.; 24 cm. ISBN: 0721636454
Notes: Includes bibliographical references and index.

Subjects: Nursing--Vocational guidance. Nursing--Social aspects. Nursing.
LC Classification: RT82 .N874 1994
Dewey Class No.: 610.73/06/9 20

Nursing, from education to practice: Rx for success / Helen Hodges ... [et al.].
Published/Created: Norwalk, Conn.: Appleton & Lange, c1988.
Related Authors: Hodges, Helen.
Description: xii, 351 p.: ill.; 23 cm. ISBN: 0838570194 (pbk.)
Notes: Includes bibliographies and index.
Subjects: Nursing--Vocational guidance. Education, Nursing. Nursing.
LC Classification: RT82 .N865 1988
Dewey Class No.: 610.73 19

Nursing's vital signs: shaping the profession for the 1990s.
Published/Created: Battle Creek, Mich.: W.K. Kellogg Foundation, 1989.
Related Authors: National Commission on Nursing Implementation Project (U.S.)
Description: 156 p.: ill.; 22 cm.
Notes: "National Commission on Nursing Implementation Project"--T.p. verso.
Subtitle from cover: A design for nursing's future from the National Commission on Nursing Implementation Project. Includes bibliographical references.
Subjects: Nursing--Vocational guidance. Nursing--Standards. Nursing audit. Nursing--standards. Nursing--trends. Nursing Audit.
LC Classification: RT82 .N88 1989

Ostner, Ilona.
Krankenpflege, ein Frauenberuf?: Bericht über eine empirische Untersuchung / Ilona Ostner; Almut Krutwa-Schott.
Published/Created: Frankfurt [Main]; New York: Campus-Verlag, 1981.
Related Authors: Krutwa-Schott, Almut.
Description: 197 p.; 21 cm. ISBN: 3593327899
Notes: Bibliography: p. 179-184.
Subjects: Nursing. Nursing--Vocational

guidance. Women--Employment. Nursing-
-Germany--History.
Series: Forschungsberichte aus dem
Sonderforschungsbereich 101
(Sozialwissenschaftliche Berufs- und
Arbeitskräfteforschung) der Universität
München
LC Classification: RT82 .O87
Dewey Class No.: 610.73/06/9 19
National Bib. No.: GFR81-A

Pinding, Maria.
Krankenpflege in unserer Gesellschaft;
Aspekte aus Praxis und Forschung. Hrsg.
von Maria Pinding. Stuttgart, F.
Published/Created: Enke, 1972.
Description: xv, 231 p. 24 cm. ISBN:
3432017529:
Notes: Includes bibliographies.
Subjects: Nursing and nursing--Social
aspects. Nursing--Vocational guidance.
LC Classification: RT42 .P56
National Bib. No.: GDB***

Pivar, William H.
Survival manual for nursing students /
William Pivar.
Published/Created: Philadelphia: Saunders,
1979.
Description: vi, 180 p.: ill.; 25 cm. ISBN:
0721672523
Notes: Includes index. Bibliography: p.
159-176.
Subjects: Nursing--Study and teaching.
Nursing students. Nursing--Vocational
guidance.
Variant Series: Saunders survival series
LC Classification: RT71 .P58
Dewey Class No.: 610.73/07/3

Professional nursing: concepts and challenges /
[edited by] Kay Kittrell Chitty.
Edition Information: 2nd ed.
Published/Created: Philadelphia: W.B.
Saunders, c1997.
Related Authors: Chitty, Kay Kittrell.
Description: xvii, 518 p.: ill.; 23 cm. ISBN:
0721668828

Notes: Includes bibliographical references
and index.
Subjects: Nursing--Vocational guidance.
Nursing--Social aspects. Nursing.
LC Classification: RT82 .P755 1997
Dewey Class No.: 610.73/069 20

Professional nursing: concepts and challenges /
[edited by] Kay Kittrell Chitty.
Published/Created: Philadelphia: Saunders,
c1993.
Related Authors: Chitty, Kay Kittrell.
Description: xxi, 474 p.: ill. (some col.); 23
cm. ISBN: 0721640613
Notes: Includes bibliographical references
and index.
Subjects: Nursing--Vocational guidance.
Nursing--Social aspects. Nursing.
LC Classification: RT82 .P755 1993
Dewey Class No.: 610.73/06/9 20

Puetz, Belinda E.
Networking for nurses / Belinda E. Puetz.
Published/Created: Rockville, Md.: Aspen
Systems Corp., 1983.
Related Authors: Shinn, Linda J.
Description: xiv, 206 p.; 24 cm. ISBN:
0894436708
Notes: "Networking for political impact"
and "Applying networking to labor
relations" by Linda J. Shinn: p. 103-163.
Includes bibliographical references and
index.
Subjects: Nurses--Employment. Nursing--
Vocational guidance. Career mobility--
Nursing texts. Interprofessional relations--
Nursing texts.
LC Classification: RT86.7 .P83 1983
Dewey Class No.: 610.73/06/9 19 C

Resource Publications, inc.
Index of opportunity in nursing.
Edition Information: 1969 ed.
Published/Created: Princeton, N.J. [1969]
Related Titles: Nursing profession. Index
of opportunity in the nursing profession.
Description: 92 p. 28 cm.
Notes: Caption title. Cover Index of

opportunity in the nursing profession.
Subjects: Nursing--United States. Nursing-
-Vocational guidance.
Variant Series: Career resource series A
Resource publication.
LC Classification: RT82 .R47
Dewey Class No.: 610.73/023

Resumes for nursing careers / The Editors of
VGM Career Books.
Edition Information: 2nd ed.
Published/Created: Chicago: VGM Career
Books, 2001.
Projected Pub. Date: 0110
Related Authors: VGM Career Horizons
(Firm)
Description: p. cm. ISBN: 0658017721
Subjects: Nurses--Employment. Résumés
(Employment) Nursing--Vocational
guidance.
Series: VGM professional resumes series
LC Classification: RT86.7 .R45 2001
Dewey Class No.: 610.73/06/9 21

Resumes for nursing careers / the editors of
VGM Career Horizons.
Published/Created: Lincolnwood, Ill.:
VGM Career Horizons, c1997.
Related Authors: VGM Career Horizons
(Firm)
Description: 151 p.; 28 cm. ISBN:
0844245240 (alk. paper)
Subjects: Nurses--Employment. Résumés
(Employment) Nursing--Vocational
guidance.
Series: VGM professional resumes series
VGM career books
LC Classification: RT86.7 .R45 1997
Dewey Class No.: 610.73/06/9 21

Robinson, Alice M.
Your future in nursing careers / by Alice
M. Robinson and Mary E. Reres.
Edition Information: Rev. ed.
Published/Created: New York: R. Rosen
Press, 1978.
Related Authors: Reres, Mary E., joint
author.

Description: xii, 113 p.: ill.; 22 cm.
Summary: Examines the history of nursing,
the variety of nursing careers, and the
educational and legal requirements for
them.
Notes: Cover A definitive study of your
future in nursing careers. Bibliography: p.
112-113.
Subjects: Nursing--Vocational guidance.
Nursing--Vocational guidance. Vocational
guidance.
Variant Series: Careers in depth; 99
LC Classification: RT82 .R56 1978
Dewey Class No.: 610.73/023

Robinson, Alice M.
Your future in nursing careers, by Alice M.
Robinson and Mary E. Reres.
Edition Information: [1st ed.]
Published/Created: New York, R. Rosen
Press [1972]
Related Authors: Reres, Mary E., joint
author.
Description: xii, 113 p. illus. 22 cm. ISBN:
0823902633
Summary: Examines the history of nursing,
the variety of nursing careers, and the
educational and legal requirements for
them.
Notes: Bibliography: p. 112-113.
Subjects: Nursing--Vocational guidance.
Nursing--Vocational guidance.
Variant Series: Careers in depth, 99
LC Classification: RT82 .R56
Dewey Class No.: 610.73/069

Rogers, Carla S.
How to get into the right nursing program /
Carla S. Rogers.
Published/Created: Lincolnwood, IL:
VGM Career Horizons, 1998.
Description: xi, 132 p.; 23 cm. ISBN:
084424192X
Subjects: Nursing schools--Admission.
Nursing--Vocational guidance.
Series: How to get into---
LC Classification: RT73 .R59 1998

Dewey Class No.: 610.73/06/9 21

Ropert, Hélène.
　　Comment on devient infirmière.
　　Published/Created: Verviers, Gérard et
　　Cie; Paris, l'Inter, 1969.
　　Related Authors: Olivier, Claire.
　　Description: 155 p. illus. (part col.) 18 cm.
　　Notes: Cover illustrated in color. At head
　　of Hélène Ropert répond aux questions de
　　Claire Olivier.
　　Subjects: Nursing--Vocational guidance.
　　Nursing--popular works.
　　Variant Series: Marabout service, 114.
　　Réussir
　　LC Classification: RT82
　　National Bib. No.: F70-1502

Ross, Carmen F.
　　Personal and vocational relationships in
　　practical nursing.
　　Published/Created: Philadelphia,
　　Lippincott [1961]
　　Description: 208 p. illus. 21 cm.
　　Notes: Includes bibliography.
　　Subjects: Practical nursing. Nursing--
　　Vocational guidance.
　　LC Classification: RT62 .R6
　　Dewey Class No.: 610.73
　　National Bib. No.: GB61-12165

Sacks, Terence J.
　　Careers in nursing / Terence J. Sacks.
　　Published/Created: Lincolnwood, Ill.:
　　VGM Career Horizons, c1998.
　　Description: vii, 117 p.; 24 cm. ISBN:
　　0844245542 (cloth) 0844245550 (pbk.)
　　Notes: Includes bibliographical references
　　(p. 81-84).
　　Subjects: Nursing--Vocational guidance.
　　Series: VGM professional careers series
　　LC Classification: RT82 .S23 1998
　　Dewey Class No.: 610.73/06/9 21

Schoolcraft, Victoria.
　　A down-to-earth approach to being a nurse
　　educator / Victoria Schoolcraft.
　　Published/Created: New York: Springer

Pub. Co., c1994.
　　Description: xiii, 206 p.; 24 cm. ISBN:
　　0826181309
　　Notes: Includes bibliographical references
　　and index.
　　Subjects: Nursing schools--Faculty.
　　Nursing--Vocational guidance. Faculty,
　　Nursing. Vocational Guidance.
　　Series: Springer series on the teaching of
　　nursing; v. 16
　　LC Classification: RT90 .S298 1994
　　Dewey Class No.: 610.73/071/1 20

Schulz, Cecilia L.
　　Professional nursing as a career.
　　Published/Created: Cambridge, Mass.,
　　Bellman Pub. Co., [1963]
　　Description: 22 p. illus. 23 cm.
　　Notes: Includes bibliography.
　　Subjects: Nursing--Vocational guidance.
　　Variant Series: Vocational and professional
　　monographs, no. 41.
　　LC Classification: HF5381 .V53 no. 41
　　1963

Searight, Mary W.
　　Your career in nursing [by] Mary W.
　　Searight.
　　Published/Created: New York, Messner
　　[1970]
　　Description: 190 p. illus., ports. 22 cm.
　　ISBN: 0671323393
　　Summary: Discusses the many types of
　　jobs for men and women in modern
　　nursing and the personal qualities and
　　academic training required.
　　Notes: Bibliography: p. 183-184.
　　Subjects: Nursing--Vocational guidance.
　　Nursing--Vocational guidance.
　　LC Classification: RT82 .S4
　　Dewey Class No.: 610.73/023

Seide, Diane.
　　Nurse power: new vistas in nursing / Diane
　　Seide.
　　Published/Created: New York: Lodestar
　　Books, c1986.
　　Description: xi, 109 p.; 22 cm. ISBN:

0525671730
Notes: Includes index. Bibliography: p. 99-
100.
Subjects: Nursing--Vocational guidance.
Career Mobility. Nursing.
LC Classification: RT82 .S45 1986
Dewey Class No.: 610.73/023 19

Strader, Marlene K.
Role transition to patient care management
/ Marlene K. Strader and Phillip J. Decker.
Published/Created: Norwalk, Conn.:
Appleton & Lange, c1995.
Related Authors: Decker, Phillip J.
Description: xxi, 506 p.: ill.; 24 cm. ISBN:
083856996X
Notes: Includes bibliographical references
and index.
Subjects: Nursing--Effect of managed care
on. Nursing--Vocational guidance. Health
planning--United States. Nursing services--
Administration--United States. Nursing.
Vocational Guidance. Delivery of Health
Care--organization & administration
United States. Nursing Services--
organization & administration.
LC Classification: RT82 .S86 1995
Dewey Class No.: 362.1/73/068 20

Swansburg, Russell C.
Strategic career planning and development
for nurses / Russell C. Swansburg, Philip
W. Swansburg.
Published/Created: Rockville, Md.: Aspen
Systems Corp., 1984.
Related Authors: Swansburg, Philip W.
Description: xii, 355 p.: forms; 24 cm.
ISBN: 0894435841
Notes: "An Aspen publication." Includes
index. Bibliography: p. 291-298.
Subjects: Nursing--Vocational guidance.
Nursing--Vocational guidance--United
States. Nursing. Career mobility.
Employment.
LC Classification: RT82 .S93 1984
Dewey Class No.: 610.73/02373 19

Vaillot, Madeleine Clémence.
Commitment to nursing; a philosophic
investigation.
Published/Created: Philadelphia,
Lippincott [1962]
Description: 276 p. illus. 24 cm.
Notes: Includes bibliography.
Subjects: Nursing--Vocational guidance.
Nursing schools.
LC Classification: RT82 .V3
Dewey Class No.: 610.73069
National Bib. No.: GB62-11881

Valiga, Theresa M.
The nurse educator in academia: strategies
for success / Theresa M. Valiga, Helen J.
Streubert.
Published/Created: New York: Springer
Pub. Co., c1991.
Related Authors: Streubert, Helen J.
Description: xiv, 226 p.; 22 cm. ISBN:
0826171508
Notes: Includes bibliographical references
and index.
Subjects: Nursing schools--Faculty.
Nursing--Vocational guidance. Education,
Nursing. Teaching.
Series: Springer series on the teaching of
nursing; v. 13
LC Classification: RT73 .V34 1990
Dewey Class No.: 610.73/0711 20

Vallano, Annette.
Careers in nursing: managing your future
in the changing world of healthcare /
Annette Vallano.
Published/Created: New York, NY: Simon
& Schuster, 1999.
Related Authors: Kaplan Educational
Centers (Firm: New York, N.Y.)
Description: 234 p.: ill.; 24 cm. ISBN:
0684852365
Notes: At head of Kaplan
Subjects: Nursing--Vocational guidance.
Nursing. Career Choice. Vocational
Guidance.
LC Classification: RT82 .V34 1999

Dewey Class No.: 610.73/06/9 21

Weiss, Madeline Olga.
    Opportunities in nursing careers, by M.
    Olga Weiss.
    Published/Created: New York, Vocational
    Guidance Manuals [c1964]
    Description: 128 p. 20 cm.
    Notes: Bibliography: p. 119-124.
    Subjects: Nursing--Vocational guidance.
    Variant Series: VGM career series, V155
    LC Classification: RT82 .W38
    Dewey Class No.: 610.73069

BIBLIOGRAPHY–JOURNALS AND MAGAZINES

AACN Clin Issues 1998 Feb;9(1):64-74
Pediatric intensive care: the parents' experience.
Meyer EC, Snelling LK, Myren-Manbeck LK.
Department of Pediatrics, Brown University School of Medicine, Providence, Rhode Island, USA.
A child's emergent admission to the pediatric intensive care unit (PICU) can strike fear and feelings of helplessness into the hearts of parents who only hours earlier had been in control of their lives. Acute critical illness seriously threatens the parents' ability to fulfill their familiar and important roles of protecting and providing for their child. The PICU setting can rapidly undermine the sense of competence, control, and stability of even the most dedicated parents. Parental stress is primarily caused by their displacement from familiar roles, the child's appearance and behavior, and difficulties in communicating with staff members. In planning interventions, these issues should be considered as well as the specific needs that parents have emphasized: accurate information, ready access to their children, and meaningful participation in their children's care. Advanced practice nurses are in an excellent position to improve delivery of psychosocial services to parents of critically ill children through direct care, acting as models of care practices and mentoring staff, staff education, policy development, and clinical research.

AACN Clin Issues 1999 Feb;10(1):127-32
Continuing education for advanced practice nurses.
Kleinpell RM.
Rush University College of Nursing, Chicago, IL 60657, USA.
Continuing education (CE) enables the advanced practice nurse (APN) to be apprised of practice issues and meet recertification requirements. Opportunities for obtaining CE program credits for APNs have expanded, yet uncertainty exists regarding specific program requirements for obtaining state and national certification. To obtain accurate information related to state requirements for CE for APNs, all 50 state boards of nursing were contacted by telephone in July 1998. Responses were received from all 50 states by telephone or facsimile transmission. This article outlines information related to CE for APNs including state renewal and national recertification requirements. Factors to consider when deciding on CE offerings in advanced practice nursing are also discussed.

AACN Clin Issues 2000 Feb;11(1):51-9
Awareness: the heart of cultural competence.
Leonard BJ, Plotnikoff GA.
Center for Spirituality and Healing, School of Nursing, University of Minnesota, Minneapolis 55455, USA.
Cultural competency in critical care is providing care to patients and their families that is compatible with their values and the traditions of their faiths. This requires awareness of one's own values and those of the healthcare system. The nurse must also

become aware of the cultural and spiritual values of patients and families. Although knowledge of many cultures is impossible, willingness to learn about, respect, and work with persons from different backgrounds is critical to providing culturally competent care. This article discusses elements essential for increasing cultural competency.

AAOHN J 1997 Nov;45(11):597-604; quiz 605-6
Psychological effects of stress from restructuring and reorganization. Assessment, intervention, and prevention strategies.
Short JD.
Department of Baccalaureate and Graduate Nursing, Eastern Kentucky University, Richmond, KY, USA.
1. Demands from the economy, market competition, and the political arena have led to restructuring, reorganization, and change in the workplace. 2. Work behaviors indicative of stress are costly to organizations. 3. Strategies for intervention and prevention should be directed at both managers and workers and can result in cost savings for the organizations. 4. A collaborative approach in which occupational health nurses work with other services inside the organization, and with community organizations and services outside the organization, is important.

Accid Emerg Nurs 1996 Jul;4(3):114-8
Comment in: Accid Emerg Nurs. 1996 Jul;4(3):109
Management of bullying and bullying in management.
Ball HC.
Bullying can be defined as 'the improper and frequent use of power to affect someone's life adversely' (Patchett 1992) or simply coercion by fear (Adams 1992). Bullying is thought to be a significant problem within the National Health Service (NHS) but this is based on anecdotal literature by Adams (1992), Turnbull (1995) and Kline (1994). There is no clear evidence as to its exact prevalence. This is not least due to the nature of the problem that inhibits reports

of the incidence of bullying. Bullying may manifest itself as a problem within a department as well as a misinformed management style. Recommendations are made to call for more awareness of the issue by research and the formation of written policies. Research based information may provide the impetus needed to introduce measures against bullying.

Accid Emerg Nurs 1996 Oct;4(4):187-9
The battered woman in the accident and emergency department.
Mortlock T.
In today's society one of the most pressing health care problems is family violence. This article focuses on female abuse and how critical care nurses need to gain awareness of their attitudes about battered women, educate themselves about the dynamics of battering and obtain the knowledge and skills needed for effective assessment and nursing intervention.

Accid Emerg Nurs 1997 Apr;5(2):81-7
Erratum in: Accid Emerg Nurs 1997 Jul;5(3):176
The work of accident and emergency nurses: Part 2. A & E maxims: making A & E work unique and special.
Sbaih L.
Manchester Metropolitan University, Department of Health Studies, UK.
An ethnomethodological study was undertaken to explore the work of Accident and Emergency (A & E) nurses; the aim of which was to analyse the ordinary, taken for granted, everyday work of those practising A & E nursing. In this second paper on the work of A & E nurses, the specific rules or maxims of nursing work in A & E are introduced. From the analysis of materials gained: fieldwork notes, observations of nurses at work and conversations, a number of maxims of A & E nursing work were identified. Maxims direct, instruct and make nurses accountable for their work and the ways in which it gets done. That is, the presence of maxims underpinning A & E nursing work ensure that A & E nursing is seen and heard as a specific type of work with its

own unique approach to talk and organization. Being aware of the maxims of A & E nursing work is not the concern of the nurse practising A & E nursing on a daily basis. Implicit and explicit reference to the maxims when talking about and doing the work provides nurses with impressions of who can do the job. Non-adherence by some nurses to the maxims of A & E nursing work often leads their colleagues to question their commitment to their choice of work setting. Maxims of A & E nursing account for the ways in which the work is seen, heard and talked about. Maxims direct the organization of work and its development within the A & E setting.

Accid Emerg Nurs 1997 Jan;5(1):16-21
Problem drinkers in accident and emergency: health promotion initiatives.
Lockhart T.
Accident & Emergency Department, Cardiff Royal Infirmary, UK.
Problems caused by excessive alcohol consumption often contribute to Accident and Emergency attendances, giving possible health promotion opportunities to this client group. These could include screening, health education (verbal or written), brief intervention and referral to alcohol services. Accident and Emergency staff rarely take these opportunities. A knowledge of alcohol problems, possible health promotion initiatives and services available alter attitudes and increase the likelihood of staff giving health promotion. Health promotion to problem drinkers should be a routine in Accident and Emergency departments.

Accid Emerg Nurs 1997 Oct;5(4):193-7
Becoming an A & E nurse.
Sbaih LC.
Manchester Metropolitan University, Department of Health Studies, UK.
This is the first of four papers which examine the work of Accident and Emergency (A & E) nurses. The descriptions in this and the following three papers have emerged from an ethnomethodological study which sought to obtain the views of what A & E nurses

believed their work to be. All are rooted in nurses' accounts of the ways in which nursing work is talked about and accomplished within the A & E setting. It should be noted that all four papers describe the ordinary rather than the extraordinary and should hold no surprises for those familiar with A & E nursing work. This first paper explores the ways in which nurses become A & E nurses, however, before descriptions can be put forward, an introduction to the study from which they have emerged needs to be made.

Accid Emerg Nurs 1998 Apr;6(2):70-4
Initial assessment: gaining impressions and 'normal cases'.
Sbaih L.
Manchester Metropolitan University, Department of Health Studies, UK.
In this third paper on the work of Accident and Emergency (A & E) nurses, the ways in which initial assessment is accomplished are described. In particular, the ability to gain an impression and use knowledge of 'normal cases' will be put forward.

Accid Emerg Nurs 1998 Apr;6(2):75-81
Resuscitation in the A & E department: can concepts of death aid decision making?
Brummell S.
Department of Acute and Critical Care, University of Sheffield, School of Nursing and Midwifery, UK.
The expectations of modern society may not recognize the limitations of technical medicine. This is particularly evident when considering the ethical problems faced by practitioners regarding the continuation or withdrawal of cardiopulmonary resuscitation within the Accident and Emergency department. This paper contends that concepts of death and our technical and cultural understanding of these must be more clearly defined and may then assist in the process of decision making. Clarifying our understanding of death, which is relevant to this clinical environment, provides us with a realistic goal for intervention. Heroic measures merely instill false hopes. A more precise delineation between cardiac arrest and

death may then guide decision making, elaborate our clinical and moral perspectives on the situation and may ease the moral burdens of this complex and sensitive aspect of practice.

Accid Emerg Nurs 1998 Jan;6(1):2-6
Initial assessment in the A & E department.
Sbaih LC.
Manchester Metropolitan University, Department of Health Studies, UK.
In this second paper on the work of Accident and Emergency (A & E) nurses, a general overview of nursing assessment in the A & E department at the point of initial nurse patient contact is put forward. This is rooted in nurses' accounts of the ways in which nursing work is talked about and accomplished within the A & E setting. Again it should be noted that this paper describes the ordinary rather than the extraordinary and should hold no surprises for those familiar with such work.

Accid Emerg Nurs 1999 Apr;7(2):106-11
Triage decision making: educational strategies.
Cioffi J.
Faculty of Health, University of Western Sydney, Hawkesbury, NSW, Australia.
Patient triage in Accident and Emergency departments requires emergency nurses to make rapid decisions based on their knowledge and experiences. The development of triage decision-making skills can be addressed through the use of simulations, 'thinking aloud' technique, reflection and the decision rules of experienced emergency nurses. Clinical educators and experienced emergency nurse mentors are encouraged to recognize that skill acquisition in triage decision making requires practice before registered nurses can engage fully in the process of triaging patients in the emergency department. It is essential to experience the process of triage decision making in order to develop an understanding of the clinical information attended to, the sequence in which the information is processed and the rules used to combine information leading to a decision on the triage category for each patient. By using triage simulations

developed from 'real triage cases' the process of decision making can be experienced by nurses. Further, if these simulations are accompanied by the collection of verbal protocols, nurses have opportunities retrospectively to explore their decision making with reflection. In addition, the presentation and use of decision rules used by experienced triage nurses can enhance the development of skills in novice triage nurses.

Adv Ren Replace Ther 1996 Jul;3(3):218-21
Nursing interventions related to vascular access infections.
Thomas-Hawkins C.
University of Pennsylvania Outpatient Dialysis Center, Philadelphia, USA.
Vascular access infection is a common cause of the loss of a vascular access. Education of both nursing staff and patients is essential for preventing vascular access infections and for treating infections early. The use of strict aseptic technique is essential when providing vascular access care. Central venous catheters require special assessment and care. Dialysis staff can have a critical role in prevention and early treatment of vascular access infections.

Age Ageing 1997 Sep;26 Suppl 2:31-5
Variation in training programmes for Resident Assessment Instrument implementation.
Bernabei R, Murphy K, Frijters D, DuPaquier JN, Gardent H.
Universita Cattolica del Sacro Cuore, Roma, Italy. md0516@mclink.it
BACKGROUND: this paper provides an overview of the Minimum Data Set/Resident Assessment Instrument (MDS/RAI) training programmes in eight countries where the system has been introduced into nursing homes. Formal education and training in the skills of assessment and care planning of nursing home personnel is reputed to be poor. In response to this problem several researchers and clinicians view MDS/RAI implementation as an opportunity to upgrade staff knowledge in care of elderly people.

RESULTS: the courses in the eight countries varied in content and length according to the different goals each interRAI researcher planned when the MDS/RAI was implemented. As expected the greatest differences in training approach were between the USA and other countries. In the USA, where the MDS/RAI was mandated for use in all nursing homes, tens of thousands of professionals had to be oriented to use the system in a relatively short period of time in order to comply with the law. The training programmes therefore tended to be very short compared with those that emerged in countries where the MDS/RAI was freely chosen and implemented.

Am J Hosp Palliat Care 1997 May-Jun;14(3):110-3
The hardiness of hospice nurses.
Hutchings D.
Hardiness is a developing concept of particular relevance and interest to nursing. Hardiness is defined as a personality construct that is an amalgam of three main elements: control, challenge and commitment. Kobasa asserts that an investment of committed energy serves to strengthen a person under stress or when faced with challenges. Hospice nurses confront a myriad of challenges associated with the rapidly changing needs of dying people and their friends and families. This author suggests that the very nature of palliative care requires mobilization of the same three constituents of hardiness, i.e., control, challenge, and commitment, blended with the key hospice elements of critical competence and compassionate care. This article considers a possible relationship between hardiness and hospice nurses, suggesting that not only are hospice nurses hardy, but that the very practice and philosophy of palliative care is predicated on a triad of control, challenge, and commitment harnessed in concert for the delivery of skilled, compassionate care to dying persons.

Am J Med 1999 May;106(5):565-73
Delirium: a symptom of how hospital care is failing older persons and a window to improve quality of hospital care.
Inouye SK, Schlesinger MJ, Lydon TJ.
Department of Internal Medicine, Yale University School of Medicine, New Haven, CT 06504, USA.
Delirium, or acute confusional state, which often results from hospital-related complications or inadequate hospital care for older patients, can serve as a marker of the quality of hospital care. By reviewing five pathways that can lead to a greater incidence of delirium--iatrogenesis, failure to recognize delirium in its early stages, attitudes toward the care of the elderly, the rapid pace and technological focus of health care, and the reduction in skilled nursing staff--we identify how future trends and cost-containment practices may exacerbate the problem. Examining delirium also provides an opportunity to improve the quality of hospital care for older persons. Interventions to reduce delirium would need to occur at the local and national levels. Local strategies would include routine cognitive assessment and the creation of systems to enhance geriatric care, such as incentives to change practice patterns, geriatric expertise, case management, and clinical pathways. National strategies might include providing education for physicians and nurses to improve the recognition of delirium and the awareness of its clinical implications, improving quality monitoring systems for delirium, and creating environments to facilitate the provision of high-quality geriatric care.

Am J Med 1999 May;106(5):565-73
Delirium: a symptom of how hospital care is failing older persons and a window to improve quality of hospital care.
Inouye SK, Schlesinger MJ, Lydon TJ.
Department of Internal Medicine, Yale University School of Medicine, New Haven, CT 06504, USA.
Delirium, or acute confusional state, which often results from hospital-related complications or inadequate hospital care for older patients, can serve as a marker of the quality of hospital care. By reviewing five pathways that can lead to a greater incidence of delirium--iatrogenesis, failure

to recognize delirium in its early stages, attitudes toward the care of the elderly, the rapid pace and technological focus of health care, and the reduction in skilled nursing staff--we identify how future trends and cost-containment practices may exacerbate the problem. Examining delirium also provides an opportunity to improve the quality of hospital care for older persons. Interventions to reduce delirium would need to occur at the local and national levels. Local strategies would include routine cognitive assessment and the creation of systems to enhance geriatric care, such as incentives to change practice patterns, geriatric expertise, case management, and clinical pathways. National strategies might include providing education for physicians and nurses to improve the recognition of delirium and the awareness of its clinical implications, improving quality monitoring systems for delirium, and creating environments to facilitate the provision of high-quality geriatric care.

Am J Nurs 1996 Sep;96(9):42-7; quiz 48
Comment in: Am J Nurs. 1996 Dec;96(12):16
Delegation are you doing it right?
Parkman CA.
Sharp Memorial Hospital, San Diego, CA, USA.

Am J Nurs 1998 Feb;98(2):26-32; quiz 33
Comment in: Am J Nurs. 1998 Jul;98(7):21
Delegation alert!
Boucher MA.
Frances Payne Bolton School of Nursing, Case Western Reserve University, Cleveland, OH, USA.

Am J Nurs 1998 Jun;98(6):34-9; quiz 39-40
Managed care: the value you bring.
Elder KN, O'Hara N, Crutcher T, Wells N, Graham C, Heflin W.
Vanderbilt University Medical Center, Nashville, TN, USA.

Am J Nurs 2001 Feb;101(2):26-31; quiz 31-2
The impact of staff nurses on the recruitment of patients.

Joseph M, Freda MC.
Albert Einstein College of Medicine, Montefiore Medical Center, Bronx, NY 10461, USA. margaretfreda@netscape.net

Anaesthesist 1997 Mar;46(3):177-85
[Palliative medicine]
[Article in German]
Klaschik E, Husebo S.
Abteilung fur Anasthesiologie, Intensivmedizin und Schmerztherapie, Malteser
Krankenhaus Bonn.
Palliative medicine has its origin in the modern hospice movement. It is based upon an integrated-care concept for seriously ill and dying patients. The first consideration of this particular form of treatment is not to prolong life, but to reach the best possible quality of a patient's remaining lifetime. Therefore, palliative medicine consists of: (1) excellent pain treatment and symptom control; (2) an integrated approach towards the psychic, social, and spiritual needs of the patient, relatives, and attending staff during the periods of illness, dying, and, after the patient's death; (3) competence in dealing with vital matters of communication and ethics; and (4) acceptance of death as a normal process. Palliative medicine clearly rejects euthanasia. Practical implementation of the idea of hospice services can be realised anywhere when taking care of seriously ill and dying patients, whether at home, in a nursing home, or in hospital. Experience shows that quite a few patients cannot be treated successfully without additional services, such as home-care services, day-care centres, in patient hospices, and palliative-care units. Up to now, severely ill tumour patients have benefited most from these services. In palliative care units an interdisciplinary team of doctors and nursing staff assisted by physiotherapists and members of psycho-social professions is taking care of and treating patients. Additional support is given by voluntary services and the integration of the patient's relatives in the caring process. Palliative medicine is the overall term for this special kind of treatment and care. In Great

Britain, Canada, and Scandinavia considerable progress has been achieved in this field, including recognition as an independent clinical discipline and the establishment of lectureships in palliative medicine.

Annu Rev Nurs Res 1994;12:95-123
Nursing workload measurement systems.
Edwardson SR, Giovannetti PB.
School of Nursing, University of Minnesota.

ANS Adv Nurs Sci 1994 Jun;16(4):42-54
Connective leadership for the 21st century: a historical perspective and future directions.
Klakovich MD.
Azusa Pacific University, California.
Health care reform, layoffs, and hospital closures have created substantial stress for both nursing leadership and nursing staff. History suggests that nursing staff and leaders have not felt closely aligned and mutually supportive. An environment that provides a means for renewal of caregivers and administrators is needed to sustain caring practice. A new leadership paradigm, connective leadership, is proposed to address the problems of the past. Connective leaders, by empowering staff at all levels, facilitate the collaboration and synergism needed in the reformed health care environment of the future.

ANZ J Surg 2001 May;71(5):285-9
Management of extravasation injuries.
Kumar RJ, Pegg SP, Kimble RM.
Burns Unit, Royal Clinic Children's Hospital, Brisbane, Queensland, Australia.
BACKGROUND: Various agents have been implicated in causing tissue necrosis after intravenous infusions have extravasated. These include solutions of calcium, potassium, bicarbonate, hypertonic dextrose, cytotoxic drugs and antibiotics. Views on management of these injuries differ, and range from a non-operative conservative approach to early debridement and grafting.
METHODS: A retrospective review was undertaken of the hospital files of patients with extravasation injuries seen in three Australian hospitals. Nine patients were identified, and their management and long-term follow up are reported.
RESULTS: Age ranged from 17 days to 60 years. Two patients received their injuries from solutions containing isotonic dextrose/saline. The other seven patients received injuries from a variety of solutions including calcium gluconate (n = 1), parenteral nutrition (n = 1), sodium bicarbonate (n = 1), immunoglobulin (n = 1), gentamicin and penicillin (n = 1), flucloxacillin (n = 1), and the chemotherapeutic agents epirubicin and cyclophosphamide (n = 1). The sites involved included the dorsum of the right foot (n = 3), the dorsum of the left foot (n = 3), the right groin (n = 1), the right hand (n = 1) and the left hand (n = 1). Four patients were managed by delayed debridement and split skin grafting, while five were treated non-operatively. Prolonged scar management was necessary in seven of the nine patients. Final results were satisfactory in all patients who received skin grafting and in all patients who were managed conservatively.
CONCLUSIONS: Management of extravasation injuries should be conservative if possible. Delayed debridement and split skin grafting is required if the area of skin loss is extensive. Scar management remains a problem. Prevention of these injuries with the education of both medical and nursing staff remains the ultimate aim.
Publication Types: Review; Review, Multicase

Arch Psychiatr Nurs 1992 Jun;6(3):163-71
Nurses as patient assault victims: an update, synthesis, and recommendations.
Lanza ML.
Nursing Service for Research, Edith Nourse Rogers Memorial Veterans Hospital, Bedford, MA 01730.
The literature documenting the incidence and reactions of nursing staff who have been assaulted by patients is increasing. Before 1980 very little work was done in the area. What did appear generally indicated that patient violence against staff

was infrequent, and on the rare occasion when it did occur the staff member was usually in some way responsible. Current research shows that assault is a serious risk factor for nurses. The incidence of assault is high and vastly underreported. Staff members experience short- and long-term emotional, social, biophysiological, and cognitive reactions to being assaulted. Interventions to help the staff victim in the recovery process are increasingly used.

Aten Primaria 1996 Jan;17(1):24-32
[Professional profile of primary health care personnel. A Delphi study]
[Article in Spanish]
Molina Duran F, Ballesteros Perez AM, Martinez Ros MT, Soto Calpe R, Sanchez Sanchez F.
Unidad Doncente de Medicina de Familia y Comunitaria de Murcia.
OBJECTIVE: To determine the professional profile of health staff (doctors, paediatricians and nurses) in primary care (PC).
DESIGN: Three simultaneous Delphi techniques (consensus method).
SETTING: Primary care.
PARTICIPANTS: 55 doctors, 45 nurses and 23 paediatricians from the whole of Spain and different fields of activity.
INTERVENTION: The filling in of three questionnaires, using the Delphi methodology.
RESULTS: The overall percentage of replies was 69.1% (first questionnaire), 70.7% (2nd) and 60.16% (3th). The PC doctor should guide in a suitable way his/her community's health problems, using the relevant diagnostic and therapeutic methods, caring for patients' all-round health, controlling the doctor-patient interview, all in collaboration with other professionals, with a planning, programming and evaluation of his/her activity and a basically community-oriented approach. The nursing professional should provide all-round care for patients, using nursing diagnostic and therapeutic methods, within a multidisciplinary team and carrying out planning, programming and evaluation of the community's health problems. The PC

paediatrician should be concerned with the prevention and treatment of the most common pathologies. He/she has a vital role to play in childrens' health education, should have the training to resolve the most common paediatric emergencies and organise his/her work within a multidisciplinary team.
CONCLUSIONS: The Delphi method is a useful technique for determining professional profiles. Paediatricians have a more sharply defined profile than doctors and nursing staff.
Publication Types: Consensus Development Conference Review

Aust Crit Care 1998 Mar;11(1):10-4
Australian nurses and device use: the ideal and the real in clinical practice.
Pelletier D, Duffield C, Mitten-Lewis S, Nagy S, Crisp J.
University of Technology, Sydney, New South Wales.
Clinical nurses use an increasing number of technological devices when providing care. While the clinical devices themselves must undergo rigorous multidimensional assessment, it is the proficiency of the user that ultimately determines the devices' efficacy. Thus, the knowledge, skills and attitudes that nurses bring to their decision-making and use of technology are crucial elements in the technology assessment process. Technological proficiency is imperative in the current climate of rapid patient throughput in complex technological environments. This paper reports some of the findings of an Australian study, using two national Delphi panels, whose primary objective was to determine the knowledge, skills and attitudes required of expert clinicians for practice in cardiac care. Panels of 28 educators and 42 cardiac nurse clinicians completed a questionnaire indicating the importance of 107 characteristics of expert cardiac practice for both the 'real' and 'ideal' worlds of practice. Comparative results will be reported for 29 items within the thematic groups. Effective use of technology, Informed decisions regarding equipment and Critical approach to the use of technology. Both panels accepted all 29

items in these three thematic groups but indicated differences in the level of agreement on the importance of items between the 'real' and 'ideal' worlds of practice. Discussion centers around those areas where improvement is needed.

Aust Crit Care 1998 Mar;11(1):10-4
Australian nurses and device use: the ideal and the real in clinical practice.
Pelletier D, Duffield C, Mitten-Lewis S, Nagy S, Crisp J.
University of Technology, Sydney, New South Wales.
Clinical nurses use an increasing number of technological devices when providing care. While the clinical devices themselves must undergo rigorous multidimensional assessment, it is the proficiency of the user that ultimately determines the devices' efficacy. Thus, the knowledge, skills and attitudes that nurses bring to their decision-making and use of technology are crucial elements in the technology assessment process. Technological proficiency is imperative in the current climate of rapid patient throughput in complex technological environments. This paper reports some of the findings of an Australian study, using two national Delphi panels, whose primary objective was to determine the knowledge, skills and attitudes required of expert clinicians for practice in cardiac care. Panels of 28 educators and 42 cardiac nurse clinicians completed a questionnaire indicating the importance of 107 characteristics of expert cardiac practice for both the 'real' and 'ideal' worlds of practice. Comparative results will be reported for 29 items within the thematic groups. Effective use of technology, Informed decisions regarding equipment and Critical approach to the use of technology. Both panels accepted all 29 items in these three thematic groups but indicated differences in the level of agreement on the importance of items between the 'real' and 'ideal' worlds of practice. Discussion centres around those areas where improvement is needed.

Aust Crit Care 1999 Sep;12(3):109-18
A review of intensive care nurse staffing

practices overseas: what lessons for Australia?
Clarke T, Mackinnon E, England K, Burr G, Fowler S, Fairservice L.
University of Sydney.
In view of market-driven health-care policies and the move to greater efficiencies within the health-care system, the cost of nursing care is being increasingly scrutinised. Different overseas practices are commonly cited as justification for changing practices within Australia. This study is based on a review of the literature on intensive care nurse staffing requirements in Australasia; specifically, New South Wales, the United States (US) and, to a lesser extent, Europe. It was found that looking to the US for cost-cutting strategies in intensive care units (ICUs) is based on a false premise: that we are comparing like with like. ICUs in the US have a different historical trajectory and culture, service wider constituencies, have technicians and unregistered personnel providing nursing care and do not provide demonstrably better outcomes or significant cost savings. Research indicates that continuous nursing care by trained professionals provides the best outcomes. If costs must be cut, technology, pharmaceuticals and laboratory tests should be targeted. Further, a greater commitment to the development of a 'progressive patient care' model in hospital planning is required, in order to establish or consolidate an intermediate level of nursing care between the ward and the ICU. Programs aiming to improve and continuously monitor patient care, such as adverse event monitoring, the prevention of unplanned extubation and facilitation of early extubation, should be instituted, as these have been shown to not only reduce ICU costs but also improve patient outcomes.
Publication Types: Review; Review Literature

Aust N Z J Ment Health Nurs 1996 Dec;5(4):153-62
Forensic psychiatric nursing: visions of social control.
Mason T, Mercer D.

Liverpool University/Ashworth Hospital Merseyside, England.
Forensic nursing is a relatively recent, and fast developing, specialization within the wider field of psychiatry. The construction of professional practice at the interface of medical and legal services reflects larger ideological shifts in the management of human difference. Central to this trend is the posited relationship between mental disorder and criminality. The expanding loci of forensic expertise, beyond traditional institutional and health service settings, calls for a critical appraisal of present and proposed provision. Focusing on the British experience, in particular, this paper outlines the historical development of treatment for disordered offenders and explores contemporary initiatives. Deployment of nursing staff in the community, police stations, law courts and prisons, as an adjunct of medicalized crime, confuses further professional care with political control. The main conclusions presented are that the encroachment of psychiatry can be understood in terms of surveillance and social control. It is essential that nurses working in this field are aware of the power/knowledge equation that frames their practice, research and education. The penetration of forensic nursing into realms of society otherwise bereft of psychiatric intervention can be seen to have a darker dimension.

AWHONN Lifelines 1998 Oct;2(5):33-7
Assessing competence. Meeting the unique needs of nurses in small rural hospitals.
Deaton BJ, Essenpreis H, Simpson KR.
Maternity Services, St. Francis Hospital in Litchfield, IL, USA.

AWHONN Lifelines 1999 Jun-Jul;3(3):41-5
Cardiopulmonary resuscitation in pregnancy. What all nurses caring for childbearing women need to know.
Luppi CJ.
Harvard University/Brigham and Women's Hospital, Boston, MA, USA.

Best Pract Benchmarking Healthc 1997 Jul-Aug;2(4):162-7

The impact of managed care on hospital nursing.
Mayer G.
Friendly Hills HealthCare Foundation, Huntington Beach, CA, USA.
There is a significant but different role for hospital staff nurses within a managed care environment. This article describes the role and reviews major areas where the staff nurse is critical in achieving positive patient outcomes that are cost-effective and efficient.

Br J Nurs 1996 Apr 11-24;5(7):400-3
Implications of transplantation surgery for theatre nurses: 1.
Clay J, Crookes PA.
Rotherham District General Hospital.
Transplant donors, although legally dead, arrive in operating theatre departments appearing no different from any other preoperative patient. Some theatre staff may not appreciate, or even be aware, that transplant donors have been certified dead before donor surgery. This article, the first of two-parts, examines the implications of organ donation surgery for the emotional and psychological wellbeing of nursing staff. Other potential problems for nursing staff, related to the process of organ retrieval, are also explored. These include the scheduling of transplant work at times when there is a poor level of skill mix, difficulties in working with unfamiliar staff and equipment, the apparent lack of 'benefit' of surgery for donor patients, and the possibility of identifying with the victims of sudden and perhaps traumatic death. The second article, to be published in the next issue, will discuss ways of ameliorating the stress associated with this work.

Br J Nurs 1996 May 9-22;5(9):552-5
Accepting the challenges of pain management.
Browne R.
Despite advances in the treatment of pain, studies reveal that hospitalized patients continue to suffer under-recognised and unrelieved pain. Several factors contribute to this problem including health-care professionals' lack of knowledge about

pain and analgesia, the inadequate use of pain assessment techniques and incomplete charting of patients' reports of pain. This article describes these challenges which must be overcome if the situation is to improve. It outlines the potential value of systematic assessment and documentation of pain so that the patient's pain is acknowledged as a unique experience. This should enable the health professional to individualize his/her approach to pain management.

Br J Nurs 1997 Dec 11-1998 Jan 7;6(22):1278-80, 1282-4
Handwashing: still a neglected practice in the clinical area.
Gilmour J, Hughes R.
Northern Area College of Nursing, Antrim, Northern, Ireland.
This article is an adaptation of the winning essay in the preregistration section of the National Board for Northern Ireland Research Awards 1996. The authors conducted a literature review of handwashing after discovering during clinical placements that, despite being well documented, handwashing is still not performed as necessary. The aim of handwashing is to remove transient microorganisms and prevent their transfer to susceptible patients. Inadequate training, lack of resources, chapped hands and poor reinforcement were identified by nurses as factors that accounted for poor handwashing. The Code of Professional Conduct states that 'the professional has a duty to promote and safeguard the interests of clients.' It is only a matter of time before major litigation occurs because of poor handwashing practice. It is concluded that all staff (trained and untrained) require regular educational updating to sustain good handwashing practices. Managers are responsible for ensuring the provision of adequate facilities and supplies of handwashing agents for all nurses in all clinical settings.

Br J Nurs 1997 Jun 12-25;6(11):607-11
Nurses' documentation of infection control precautions: 1.
Finn L.

Communicable Disease Control, Dorset Health Authority, Victoria House, Ferndown.
Inadequate nursing records may contribute to untoward incidents and yet advised precautions for the control of infection can be poorly documented. The infection control nurse must promote a safe environment for the patient and ensure that an effective control policy is carried out. The literature suggests that nurses may lack the necessary knowledge and skills with which to assess, plan and evaluate appropriate care for safe infection control. This article, the first of two parts, discusses these issues together with various strategies at the infection control nurse's disposal that may influence nursing practice and the documentation of care.
Publication Types: Review; Review Literature

Br J Nurs 1997 Nov 27-Dec 10;6(21):1218-20, 1222, 1224-8
Intravenous therapy: current practice and nursing concerns.
Campbell T, Lunn D.
Dorset Cancer Centre.
The field of intravenous (i.v.) therapy has been subject to major change, with increasing numbers of nurses taking on the high profile, technical aspects of care. The transfer of previously medicalized tasks such as cannulation has been welcomed by nurses who are keen to develop practical skills in order to embrace the concept of holistic patient care. This literature review aims to clarify the role of the nurse in i.v. therapy, exploring cannulation as a specific issue. Legal and professional aspects are discussed in terms of extended/expanded practice and practical aspects in terms of i.v. access and maintenance. Discussion focuses on a team approach to the management of i.v. therapy. Finally, the nursing process is applied to an i.v. therapy scenario. Exploration of the nursing issues enables practitioners to justify the expansion of individual practice in order to deliver holistic care and improve standards of service. The review concludes that nurses cannot afford to lose sight of the caring component of their role as a result

of immersion in the culture of technical skill acquisition.

Br J Nurs 1998 Apr 9-22;7(7):388-92
Stroke 2: expanding the nurse's role in stroke rehabilitation.
Nolan M, Nolan J.
School of Nursing and Midwifery, University of Sheffield.
This article, the second of two considering the nurse's role in stroke rehabilitation, focuses on potential nursing contributions in a number of areas. There is scope, particularly in the community, to develop a far greater nursing role in both the acute and the postacute phases of rehabilitation. However, nurses often have ambivalent attitudes towards rehabilitation--seeing acute care as more prestigious and important. Such attitudes are developed and reinforced in basic training which gives relatively little emphasis to chronic illness.

Br J Nurs 1998 Jun 11-24;7(11):658-62
Does the specialist nurse enhance or deskill the general nurse?
Marshall Z, Luffingham N.
Department of Anaesthetics, Pain Relief, University Hospital Lewisham, London.
Much conflict and confusion surrounds the title and role of the specialist nurse, leading in some instances to disharmony between general and specialist nurses. It has been suggested that too many highly specialized nurses in a general area may lead to a deskilled workforce and fragmented care. Attempts to define the key concepts of specialist practice as described by the UKCC has resulted in elitism, conflict and abuse of the title. One suggestion to eliminate this conflict is for specialist nurses to achieve key competencies that encompass the role of the clinical expert. These key competencies should be devised by specialist nurses, in the absence of national guidelines, and be agreed by employers. They should incorporate the key roles of: change agent, expert clinician, educator, researcher and coordinator. It is contended that if all concerned have a clearer definition of the title, role and what is expected from the specialist nurse then this will result in reduced conflict and improved quality of care.

Br J Nurs 1998 May 28-Jun 10;7(10):571-4, 576 passim
Moving and handling practice in neuro-disability nursing.
Billin SL.
Department, Royal Hospital for Neuro-disability, West Hill, Putney, London.
This article examines the challenge of implementing a safer handling policy in an environment which caters for the needs of people who have complex and profound disability. It explores how a moving and handling educational strategy has been developed and the effectiveness of the strategies employed. The impact of changing practice at ward level and the difficulties encountered will be discussed in light of the patients' complex needs. The effects of the strategy are outlined with regard to accident reporting and the impact of legislation regarding moving and handling in an environment where patients' needs have to be balanced with staff safety are considered.

Br J Nurs 1998 Nov 26-Dec 9;7(21):1318-22
Personal, professional and practice development: clinical supervision.
Cutcliffe JR, Burns J.
Sheffield University.
This article investigates current research concerns in relation to clinical supervision and offers a rationale for using case studies as a means of evaluation. Three case studies are used to illustrate how development and growth can occur as a result of clinical supervision. The use of case studies as a means of evaluation is analysed. Case studies provide unique insights into the dynamics and processes of clinical supervision. Any improvement in practice ought to bring about improvements in client care, thus case studies can add to the accumulating, qualitative data that support the link between clinical supervision and improved client care. This article recommends that more case studies should be carried out and that the findings are compiled on a centralized database in order that evidence

supporting the widespread use of clinical supervision is readily accessible.

Br J Nurs 1998 Sep 10-23;7(16):946-8, 950, 952
Three major issues in infection control.
Perry C.
Southmead Health Services (NHS) Trust.
In considering the three major issues in infection control the author decided upon education and empowerment, community practices, and research availability and application as they span a range of infection control practices and healthcare settings. Education and empowerment of staff is needed to ensure safe practice. This requires collaboration between education providers and infection control personnel and should be available to all disciplines of staff. Infection control needs to be seamless across the primary and secondary care interface and must include infection prevention advice to the population in general. Evidence relating to infection control is either lacking or not achievable. When it is available, it is not always implemented because of lack of resources.

Br J Nurs 1999 Apr 22-Mar 12;8(8):500-4
Tracheostomy care: tracheal suctioning and humidification.
Buglass E.
Ear, Nose and Throat/Head and Neck Unit, Queen Elizabeth Hospital, Birmingham.
Tracheostomy care is a complex nursing activity and has many potential complications. However, aspects of tracheostomy care appear to be carried out without uniformity and with some confusion as to correct techniques, especially outside the ear, nose and throat and intensive care environments. Some aspects of the literature appear contradictory, leaving nurses to make individual judgments about correct procedures. It is the nurse who is accountable for the care given; therefore, with the wealth of evidence available, it is important that the nurse is adequately trained and fully competent in the care of a patient with a tracheostomy. This article discusses particular aspects of tracheostomy care: assessment; tracheal

suctioning; suction pressure; suction catheters; and humidity.

Br J Nurs 1999 Apr 22-Mar 12;8(8):524-9
Understanding clinical supervision from a nursing perspective.
Sloan G.
Cognitive Behavioural Psychotherapy, Consulting and Clinical Psychology Services, Ayrshire and Arran Community Healthcare Trust, Ayr.
During the last 10 years there has been an increase in the amount of nursing literature dealing with clinical supervision. As a result, there has been a gradual growth in the use of clinical supervision to provide support, increase clinical competence and improve client care. Unfortunately, there has not been a comparable increase in research and as a result the amount of empirical knowledge is minimal. This article will discuss the key empirical studies that have focused on identifying the outcomes of supervision and isolating the characteristics that make a good clinical supervisor. Recommendations for practice and research will be suggested.
Publication Types: Review; Review Literature

Br J Nurs 1999 Apr 8-21;8(7):426-31
A practical guide to venepuncture and management of complications.
Campbell H, Carrington M, Limber C.
Practice Development Team, York District Hospital.
For years many nurses have felt that if they had the ability to perform skills such as venepuncture they would be able to provide a more holistic and efficient service. The culture in which nurses and doctors have traditionally worked has often made it difficult for nurses to become competent at such skills. However, the boundaries of medical and nursing roles have started to change and a culture of shared roles is emerging which has many benefits for patients, medical staff and nursing staff. This article provides a practical guide to venepuncture. It highlights the structure of a vein and the veins that are suitable for venepuncture. It also addresses the prevention and

management of potential complications.

Br J Nurs 1999 Feb 11-24;8(3):165-8
Triage in accident and emergency. 2:
Educational requirements.
Wilkinson RA.
Accident and Emergency Department,
Torbay Hospital, Torquay.
The first article in this two-part series on
the review of the concept of triage (Vol
8(2): 86-102) examined the areas of
waiting times, patient satisfaction and the
difficulty of trying to implement universal
standards into accident and emergency
(A&E) departments because of their
varying infrastructures. This article aims to
identify the educational requirements
needed to become a triage nurse. Indeed,
none of the reviewed literature explicitly
addresses this issue. Educational literature
tends to focus on the scientific aspect of
practice rather than acknowledging that art,
where interactions between the nurse and
patient are essentially social acts that can
never be accounted for by science, is also
an inherent part of nursing practice. This
article also investigates and analyses the
use of research methods utilized to
investigate triage and suggests that a re-
evaluation of these methods is needed if
the true effects of triage are to be
ascertained.

Br J Nurs 1999 Jul 8-21;8(13):866-70
Learning disabilities: supporting nurses in
delivering primary care.
Stanley R.
Faculty of Healthcare Sciences, Kingston
University, London.
This article introduces an educational
project supported by The Queen's Nursing
Institute and sponsored by the
Hertfordshire Nursing Trust. It reports on
the initial results from a literature review
and its implications for nursing. There is
broad acknowledgement of a problem in
the delivery of primary care nursing for
people with a learning disability, but little
consensus on how to move either medical
or nursing practice forward. It was
proposed, therefore, to systematically
assess the learning needs of nurses
delivering primary care and to develop an

evaluated methodology for responding to
those needs. A comprehensive literature
review was undertaken. Three consistent
themes emerged: knowledge and training
needs; role definitions and liaison; and
clinical issues. Implications for nursing,
and the future development of the project
are considered.

Br J Nurs 1999 Jun 10-23;8(11):716-20
Importance of handwashing in the
prevention of cross-infection.
Parker LJ.
Scunthorpe General Hospital.
Although the importance of handwashing
is routinely acknowledged, a religious
application of this practice still does not
exist. Discussion in modern medicine on
the subject of handwashing always states
that it is the single most important factor in
preventing hospital-acquired infection.
This article continues the series on
infection control and practical procedures
by looking at the evidence that supports the
above statement and discusses various
handwashing methods and how to increase
compliance to handwashing in the
healthcare setting.

Br J Nurs 1999 May 27-Jun 9;8(10):653-6
Prison health care: work environment and
the nursing role.
Norman A, Parrish A.
This article, the first in a new series on
prison nursing, gives an overview of the
world of prison nursing and the
environmental factors that make it so
different from other types of nursing. It
welcomes the recommendation in the
report 'Patient or Prisoner: A New Strategy
for Health Care in Prisons' (HM Chief
Inspector of Prisons for England and
Wales, 1996) that the NHS should be
responsible for providing health care for
prisoners and the recent publication of the
report of the Joint Prison Service/NHS
Executive Working Group 'Future
Organization of Prison health Care'
(Department of Health, 1999), which
endorses a formal partnership between the
NHS and prison service. The article
highlights the benefits that this will have
for prison nurses who often feel

professionally isolated. The role of the nurse working in the prison healthcare environment is outlined. The work of prison nurses differs from the role of nurses working in other healthcare situations as it is controlled by environmental factors associated with regimes, security and the prison culture. However, changes are taking place and a closer link with local services is envisaged. These changes are an excellent opportunity for nurses and nursing to establish a clear role in prisons and to develop further healthcare standards in the prison service.

Br J Nurs 1999 Oct 14-27;8(18):1212-4
Erratum in: Br J Nurs 1999 Dec 9-2000 Jan 12;8(22):followi
Infection control: public health, clinical effectiveness and education.
Gallagher R.
Infection Control Department, Royal United Hospital, Coombe Park, Bath.
In this article the author discusses three main issues in infection control: the development of clinical effectiveness, education and public health. Present day infection control practice is based on principles put forward by Florence Nightingale over 100 years ago. Despite medical advances, hospital-acquired infection remains a major cause of morbidity and mortality. Further research is required to assess how effective present day infection control activities and policies are in reducing the spread of infection. The success of implementing evidence-based practice relies on multidisciplinary, user-friendly educational initiatives. It is imperative that community practitioners are involved in the promotion of infection control. Greater public awareness of infectious agents and the importance of basic hygiene will ensure that infection control cannot remain the exclusive property of hospitals, but must extend to all areas of public health.

Br J Nurs 2000 Jan 13-26;9(1):43-7
Universal precautions: improving the knowledge of trained nurses.
Roberts C.
Department of Public Health Medicine,

North Wales Health Authority, Mold.
Universal precautions relate to the management of blood-borne viruses such as human immunodeficiency virus (HIV) and hepatitis B and C. Advice on the transmission of blood-borne viruses and the precautionary measures used to reduce or eliminate cross-infection have been addressed by national and professional bodies. There is a significant amount of research which assesses trained nurses' knowledge of universal precautions and includes understanding of the transmission routes of blood-borne viruses and the measures required to prevent cross-infection. However, the majority of the literature indicates an incomplete knowledge among trained nurses of the principles and application of universal precautions. The ability of the trained nurse to fulfil his/her role as health educator, teacher and therefore effective infection control practitioner is questioned by the literature. This article discusses the role of education in improving the knowledge of trained nurses and considers the implementation of in-service training and preregistration education.
Publication Types: Review; Review Literature Review, Tutorial

Br J Nurs 2000 Jan 27-Feb 9;9(2):82-6
Handwashing facilities in the clinical area: a literature review.
Ward D.
Huddersfield NHS Trust, Princess Royal Community Health Centre.
Handwashing is without doubt the most important intervention in the control of cross-infection. However, many healthcare staff do not comply with the procedure. One of the factors that contributes towards this is a lack of adequate and appropriate handwashing facilities. This article looks at the literature relating to handwashing and identifies what adequate and appropriate facilities actually are, with recommended standards for clinical areas. It concludes by highlighting that a greater commitment is needed from managers in this area in order to improve compliance with handwashing and therefore reduce infection rates.
Publication Types: Review; Review

Literature

Br J Nurs 2000 Mar 9-22;9(5):260-6
Nurse assessment of oral health: a review of practice and education.
White R. richard@medicalwriter.co.uk
The assessment of oral health status and related care of patients is a largely neglected area of nursing practice. With the notable exceptions of high-risk patient groups, such as those receiving chemotherapy in neonatal and intensive care units, and in terminal care, few patients enjoy regular, formal, oral assessments and care. Such interventions--nurse administered oral hygiene--should not be reserved only for high-risk groups but ideally be provided to all patients, whether in hospital or in the community, as they can reveal signs and symptoms of oral disease, manifestations of systemic disease, drug side-effects, or trauma; they may also provide important diagnostic clues. This article sets out to emphasize the need for nurse education in oral health care and provides a literature review and introduction to common oral health problems. It also sets out to establish the rationale for assessment in all contexts of patient care.
Publication Types: Review; Review Literature

Br J Nurs 2000 Mar 9-22;9(5):267-71
Implementing evidence-based practice in infection control.
Ward D.
Huddersfield NHS Trust, Princess Royal Community Health Centre.
Evidence-based practice is seen as a way of providing more effective health care and is considered to be vital in the current healthcare climate. However, in many areas of practice, and specifically in infection control, there is often little or no evidence to back or refute certain practices. This article looks at ritualistic practices, interventions with indirect evidence to support them and practices with overwhelming evidence in their favour which are not always followed. It is concluded that nurses need to integrate the best available evidence with clinical judgment and ensure that available evidence is disseminated appropriately.

Br J Nurs 2000Jun 8-21;9(11):724-9
Self-assessment and the concept of the lifelong learning nurse.
Gopee N.
Coventry University, School of Health and Social Sciences, Gulson Campus, Coventry.
Nurses appear to be taking an increasing interest in the concepts of lifelong learning, learning organization and a learning society. With expanding roles and their direct relevance to clinicians' different clinical grades and capacities, lifelong learning becomes an essential component in the achievement of clinical expertize. Lifelong learning is based on the self-assessment of clinical knowledge and competence. However, there are advantages as well as possible problems with both peer and self-assessments, and therefore further development and research is required.
Publication Types: Review; Review Literature

Br J Perioper Nurs 2000 Aug;10(8):412-6
A train of events?
Waller O, Waller F.
Royal Cornwall Hospitals Trust, Cornwall.
What sort of relationship do you have with your Sterile Services Department? Do you know what goes on in that department? Do their staff know what goes on in your department? In making a strong case for recognised training in Sterile Services, Olivia and Frank Waller see an exchange of experiences between operating theatres and SSD as a valuable part of the learning process. Too often separate departments only contact each other when things go wrong. The authors quote a damning judgement from an enquiry following the death of five patients: a powerful reminder of the fact that perioperative care gives only one chance to get it right. Just because you work in theatre does not mean you can ignore or take for granted those departments on which you rely for supplies and services. Get involved, find out and understand what they can do for you and

what you can do for them.

Br J Perioper Nurs 2000 Aug;10(8):421-7
Using the Internet to enhance evidence-based practice.
Orson J.
Princess Alexandra Hospital, Harlow Essex.
Evidence-based healthcare requires reliable and validated research findings to aid improved clinical practice. The Internet, with its growing medical resources, is an invaluable tool for busy healthcare workers. However, as more material becomes available on the web, the quality and reliability of various information sites is a worry for many practitioners. The ability to evaluate web sites is becoming increasingly important and as a novice user, I was interested to discover the extent to which the Internet could assist me researching a specific topic. This article describes the process of conducting an Internet search, on a topic relevant to theatre nursing, and considers how the resources might best be evaluated.

Br J Perioper Nurs 2000 Jan;10(1):30-3
Lifeskills training. You've read the books ... now it's time to apply it to life!
Brown H.
University Hospital of Wales, Cardiff.

Br J Theatre Nurs 1997 Jul;7(4):19-24
Meeting the informational needs of patients in a day surgery setting—an exploratory level study.
Reid JH.
Institute of Health and Community Studies, Bournemouth University.
This exploratory level study attempts to identify if nurses employed in a day surgery unit of a small district general hospital assess the individual informational needs of patients in their care. Data was gathered by questionnaire, highlighting a range of significant issues, which the report concludes, produces scope for future enquiry, if day surgery is to continue to accelerate toward projected purchasing and planning targets (DoH 1996), but retain a commitment to a quality assurance agenda.

Br J Theatre Nurs 1998 Apr;8(1):21-7
Educational preparation of nurses to meet the needs of human immunodeficiency virus (HIV) infected patients.
Vials JM.
School of Nursing and Midwifery, University of Wolverhampton.

Br J Theatre Nurs 1999 Aug;9(8):351-8
Parents in recovery areas: a review of the literature.
Melody A.

Br J Theatre Nurs 1999 Jul;9(7):303-8
Introducing clinical supervision into the perioperative environment.
Smith D.

Br J Theatre Nurs 1999 Nov;9(11):521-30
Organ donation--a review of the literature.
Bothamley J.
Sheffield Northern General Hospital Trust.
Organ harvesting is part of the practice of many perioperative nurses in general hospitals. It is difficult to treat as just another case because the outcome is so different to other surgery, and brings a much more intense level of emotional involvement. Add to this the fact that organ harvesting often takes place outside 'normal' working hours, and that the staff providing facilities for donation are left with the body and the mess, it is evident that both the issue and the perioperative nurse's part in this practice require some special attention. This is the first of three excellent articles by Janet Bothamley, based on her wide ranging review of the literature covering theatre nurses' perceptions of organ retrieval. Consent and patients' rights, and brain stem death, will be dealt with in the subsequent articles.
Publication Types: Review; Review Literature

Can J Cardiovasc Nurs 1997;8(1):17-23
The role of the nurse with families of patients in ICU: the nurses' perspective.
Fox S, Jeffrey J.
School of Nursing, University of Windsor, Ontario.
Although nurses are often charged with the responsibility of helping families cope with

the stress that results when a loved one is hospitalized in a critical care unit, there is little research investigating how critical care nurses perceive their role with families. The objectives of this study were to (a) describe critical care nurses' role expectations and perceived role performance with respect to patients' families, and (b) describe the relationship between nurses' role expectations and their perceived role performance. Forty-seven nurses were surveyed in this descriptive, correlational study. There was a moderately strong correlation ($r = .60$, $p < .0001$) between role expectations and role performance. However, family-focused interventions requiring less time and less intense communication skills were performed more often than those requiring more time and greater skill in communication. Thus, certain family needs may be met inconsistently due to varied perceptions among nurses regarding their responsibility to families. The findings are discussed in relation to concepts from role theory.
Publication Types: Review; Review Literature

Can J Nurs Adm 1997 Jan-Feb;10(1):24-44
The answer is ...., now what was the question? Applying alternative approaches to estimating nurse requirements.
Lavis JN, Birch S.
Division of Health Policy Research and Education, Harvard University, Boston, Massachusetts, USA.

Can J Nurs Adm 1997 Jan-Feb;10(1):45-58
The futility of utility: barriers to the development of nursing human resource policies for Ontario.
Donner G.
Faculty of Nursing, University of Toronto, ON.

Can J Nurs Adm 1997 Jan-Feb;10(1):59-68
New nursing graduates: a key factor in nursing supply.
Park C, Hughes L.
The Canadian nursing education system is the most significant contributor to the country's supply of registered nurses. This article provides current data on the numbers of nursing graduates produced in each province in 1994. The authors highlight some of the differences in the numbers produced and use the national average of new graduates as the percentage of the population of Canada as one method to arrive at the numbers of new graduates per year which each province could attempt to produce. This article provides a national perspective on current and future nursing human resources and will assist nursing administrators in their staffing plans related to registered nurses.

Can J Nurs Adm 1997 Jan-Feb;10(1):7-23
Back to the future: a framework for estimating health-care human resource requirements.
Markham B, Birch S.
Centre for Health Economics and Policy Analysis (CHEPA), McMaster University, Hamilton, Ontario.

Can Nurse 1997 Aug;93(7):38-41
Minimizing transfer injuries.
Goodridge D, Laurila B.
Riverview Health Centre, Winnipeg, Manitoba.
Publication Types: Review; Review Literature

Can Nurse 1998 Nov;94(10):36-9
Negotiation. A skill for nurses.
Hrinkanic J.
As cutbacks and health care reform bring changes to nurses' roles and health care structures, conflict almost invariably arises. Clashes stem from unclear expectations about new roles, poor communication between management and staff, a lack of clear jurisdiction over changing responsibilities, personal differences in approaches to nursing and conflicting interests as different departments struggle to maintain their share of the health care dollar. The friction could be at the individual or the group level; it might exist between shifts of nurses, between nurses and their managers, or between nurse managers and other administration. In all cases, you, the nurse, are the one who must

deal with it.

Can Nurse 1999 Nov;95(10):36-9
Boning up on i.v. push.
Power L.
Health Care Corporation of St. John's,
Newfoundland.

Can Oper Room Nurs J 2000 Jun;18(2):26-30
Expanding the role of the perioperative
educator.
Panneton Y.
Montreal Neurological Hospital, Montreal,
Quebec.
Perioperative educators mostly conduct
orientation, in service and continuing
education to perioperative staff. Their role
can be expanded to improve the quality
and efficiency of perioperative care. To
this end, an organizational communication
model can be used to identify weaknesses
and guide intervention. To be effective
with this approach, perioperative educators
have to work closely with perioperative
managers.

Can Oper Room Nurs J 2000 Mar;18(1):14-9
Is the role of circulating in an OR within
the scope of practice for the RPN?
Christiansen K.
St. Joseph's Health Centre, London,
Ontario.
Role Clarity was a focal point for
discussion by the St. Joseph's Health
Centre (SJHC) OR Practice Council. The
question: "Is the role of circulating within
the scope of practice for the Registered
Practical Nurse (RPN)?" was tabled.
Practice Council respectfully and
systematically problem solved this
question, considering factors as outlined in
the Decision Guide for determining the
Appropriate Category of Care Provider,
issued by the College of Nurses of Ontario
in March 1997. The question was analysed
and all involved parties reached consensus.
A decision followed demonstrating that the
role of the circulating nurse exceeds the
scope of practice for the RPN. The RPN
cannot fulfil the role in its entirety. This
decision resulted in a change of practice at
SJHC.
Publication Types: Consensus

Development Conference Review

Clin Lab Manage Rev 1999 Nov-
Dec;13(6):341-50
Quality assurance, practical management,
and outcomes of point-of-care testing:
laboratory perspectives, Part I.
Nichols JH, Poe SS.
Johns Hopkins University School of
Medicine, USA.
Pathologists and nurses have only recently
cooperated in point-of-care testing
(POCT), after accreditation organizations
recommended that the laboratories take
responsibility for managing the quality of
patient-care testing conducted at the
bedside. Laboratories are charged with
ensuring that patient-care tests generate
comparable results, regardless of the
location or method. Many home testing
devices, when used in hospitals,
physicians' office laboratories, and mobile
nursing practices, have presented technical
and operational issues that were not
foreseen from home use. These problems
arise from a number of factors: the way the
devices are used, the patient population,
and even differences in sample type. Thus,
to be successful, management of POCT in
the health-care environment requires
interdisciplinary cooperation of clinical
nursing staff and laboratory staff. The
article identifies problems in POCT,
describes some solutions, and examines
how well these solutions have worked from
a laboratory perspective.

Clin Nurs Res 1997 May;6(2):142-55
Gastric decompression in adult patients.
Survey of nursing practice.
Schmieding NJ, Waldman RC.
College of Nursing, University of Rhode
Island, USA.
Using a 62-item investigator-developed
mailed questionnaire, this descriptive study
of 350 randomly selected staff nurses
sought to identify variations in practices in
the care of patients with nasogastric tubes.
Reported here are the results on the 15
questionnaire items related to the use of
nasogastric tubes for gastric
decompression. Results show that practice
is not always consistent with published

research; additionally, there are areas of practice for which no research was found. Subjects' responses by age, education, and amount of experience showed marked frequency variations on several items, as did employment in teaching versus community hospitals. Results have implications for nursing educators in clinical agencies and nursing schools. Publication Types: Review; Review Literature

Clin Nurse Spec 1996 Mar;10(2):58-62
Expanding collaborative CNS efforts for research utilization.
Ohman KA.

Clin Nurse Spec 1997 Jul;11(4):169-73
Two graduating master's students struggle to find meaning.
McMyler ET, Miller DJ.
Winona State University, Rochester, Minnesota, USA.
This article was initiated to help two graduating Master's students learn what might be expected of them upon graduation. The purpose of this article is to provide insight from reviewing the current literature on clinical nurse specialist's (CNS's) characteristics. The authors believe that this information is especially useful for graduate CNS students and helpful for those who currently hold CNS positions. Based on a literature review, the article categorizes descriptions of the characteristics of the CNS role as perceived by the CNS, management, staff nurses, and physicians. Within the identified perceptions of each group were the following similarly common CNS role components: (a) clinical practice, (b) education, (c) administration, (d) research, and (e) consultation. The key to congruent expectations and understanding of the CNS role is clear communication between the members of each group. Without this communication, the common result is ambiguity, conflict, and frustration.

Clin Sports Med 1999 Oct;18(4):927-39, viii
Complications of foot and ankle surgery.
McAllister JL, Thordarson DB.
Department of Orthopaedic Surgery,

University of Southern California School of Medicine, Los Angeles, USA.
Surgery of the foot and ankle encompasses many pathologic entities, each with its own pitfalls. Some complications can be prevented through accurate diagnosis, careful patient selection, appropriate selection of surgical procedure, and thorough performance of surgical technique. Although they may arise from systemic events, immediate complications also can be diminished by training operating room personnel and nursing staff.

Collegian 1998 Jul;5(3):24-7
Evidence-based practice: an idea whose time has come.
Roberts KL.
School of Health Sciences, N.T. University.
This paper defines evidence-based practice, gives a brief history of EBP, addresses nurses' current usage of research, briefly examines the need for evidence-based practice, then addresses what evidence-based practice will mean to the profession. It is concluded that at present Australian nursing is in a stage of pre-evidence-based practice in which most Australian nurses neither read research nor apply research findings to practice. However, a demand for evidence-based practice will likely encourage nurses to use research in practice. Finally, professional strategies will be developed to encourage the introduction and evaluation of evidence-based nursing practice.

Collegian 1998 Jul;5(3):24-7
Evidence-based practice: an idea whose time has come.
Roberts KL.
School of Health Sciences, N.T. University.
This paper defines evidence-based practice, gives a brief history of EBP, addresses nurses' current usage of research, briefly examines the need for evidence-based practice, then addresses what evidence-based practice will mean to the profession. It is concluded that at present Australian nursing is in a stage of pre-

evidence-based practice in which most Australian nurses neither read research nor apply research findings to practice. However, a demand for evidence-based practice will likely encourage nurses to use research in practice. Finally, professional strategies will be developed to encourage the introduction and evaluation of evidence-based nursing practice.

Contemp Nurse 1996 Mar;5(1):28-35
Storytelling: a teaching-learning technique.
Geanellos R.
Nurses' stories, arising from the practice world, reconstruct the essence of experience as lived and provide vehicles for learning about nursing. The learning process is forwarded by combining storytelling and reflection. Reflection represents an active, purposive, contemplative and deliberative approach to learning through which learners create meaning from the learning experience. The combination of storytelling and reflection allows the creation of links between the materials at hand and prior and future learning. As a teaching-learning technique storytelling engages learners; organizes information; allows exploration of shared lived experiences without the demands, responsibilities and consequences of practice; facilitates remembering; enhances discussion, problem posing and problem solving; and aids understanding of what it is to nurse and to be a nurse.

Contemp Nurse 1999 Sep;8(3):57-64
Doing more with less in nursing work: a review of the literature.
Bradley C.
Centre for Research into Nursing and Health Care, Faculty of Nursing, University of South Australia.
The paper explores the literature on changes in nursing work. It examines the suggestion that changes in work practices are management responses to cost cutting imperatives. Nursing labour force issues such as staffing roles and staffing mix, the push for flexibility in the workforce and casualisation are discussed. The paper concludes that given the rise of casual work in the general Australian workforce, research needs to be conducted on the extent of casualisation of nursing, and the implications this may have for nursing practice, professional development and on the nursing labour market.

Crit Care Med 2001 Feb;29(2 Suppl):N26-33
The family conference as a focus to improve communication about end-of-life care in the intensive care unit: opportunities for improvement.
Curtis JR, Patrick DL, Shannon SE, Treece PD, Engelberg RA, Rubenfeld GD.
Division of Pulmonary and Critical Care Medicine, School of Medicine, University of Washington, Seattle, WA, USA.
The intensive care unit (ICU) represents a hospital setting in which death and discussion about end-of-life care are common, yet these conversations are often difficult. Such difficulties arise, in part, because a family may be facing an unexpected poor prognosis associated with an acute illness or exacerbation and, in part, because the ICU orientation is one of saving lives. Understanding and improving communication about end-of-life care between clinicians and families in the ICU is an important focus for improving the quality of care in the ICU. This communication often occurs in the "family conference" attended by several family members and members of the ICU team, including physicians, nurses, and social workers. In this article, we review the importance of communication about end-of-life care during the family conference and make specific recommendations for physicians and nurses interested in improving the quality of their communication about end-of-life care with family members. Because excellent end-of-life care is an important part of high-quality intensive care, ICU clinicians should approach the family conference with the same care and planning that they approach other ICU procedures. This article outlines specific steps that may facilitate good communication about end-of-life care in the ICU before, during, and after the conference. The article also provides direction for the future to improve physician-family and nurse-family

communication about end-of-life care in the ICU and a research agenda to improve this communication. Research to examine and improve communication about end-of-life care in the ICU must proceed in conjunction with ongoing empiric efforts to improve the quality of care we provide to patients who die during or shortly after a stay in the ICU.

Crit Care Nurs Clin North Am 1996 Dec;8(4):441-50
Maintaining competence and competency in the care of the intra-aortic balloon pump patient.
Quaal SJ.
Department of Veterans Affairs Medical Center, Salt Lake City, Utah, USA.
Care of the IABP patient requires specialized knowledge and skill. Two methods exist for verifying the nurse's ability to safely care for this patient population. Competence and competency testing approach this task from two different aspects; the former assesses the nurse's potential knowledge and skills and later verifies the nurse's ability to perform and apply knowledge, skill, and standards of care in an actual "mock run" situation. Both aspects should be included in an IABP training program.

Crit Care Nurs Clin North Am 1997 Mar;9(1):123-8
Experiences of a nursing ethics forum. Case studies and outcomes.
Bjarnason D, Prevost S, Carter M.
Department of Medical/Surgical Nursing, University of Texas Medical Branch at Galveston, USA.
Nursing staff members should need few rules and should focus on using critical thinking to guide nursing practice and care. Nurses are decision makers participating in collaborative practice. A high degree of professionalism, responsibility, and accountability is expected. We feel that this program has succeeded not only in meeting the mission and vision of the department of nursing but also that of the hospital. It also has developed to promote the philosophy that nurses must be committed to providing excellence in patient care. In addition to developing this group concept as a model, our intention is to assist staff members with the continued expansion of the group and its tenets. As Uustal asserted, the knowledge of ethical theories and principles can stimulate the nurse's thinking, and ethical decision making can offer direction; however, only you can make ethical decisions. We hope to continue the development of clinical, ethical decision-making skills and to promote the value of this program to the ongoing growth and development of professionalism in nursing.

Crit Care Nurs Clin North Am 1998 Jun;10(2):219-33
Continuous venous to venous hemofiltration. Implementing and maintaining a program: examples and alternatives.
Craig M.
Patient Care Services, University of California Davis Medical Center, Sacramento, USA.

Crit Care Nurs Clin North Am 1998 Sep;10(3):259-66
Transitioning the critical care nurse from ICU to high-tech homecare.
Newell M.
Managed Care Consultants, Merchantville, New Jersey, USA.
Critical care nurses are in a good position to take advantage of the changes in health care. They can build a career that will be on the cutting edge of the changes in technology and care delivery if they are willing to learn some new skills and practice in a more autonomous environment. Nurses who are new to the homecare setting need to know more about insurance systems, diagnosis coding, and outcomes tools and prepare themselves for the rapid growth of computer assisted technologies that are being introduced into the practice of homecare. They also need to take the whole continuum of care into consideration when planning care for patients in the home and to be aware of community and family supports that can enhance the patient's health related quality

of life.

Crit Care Nurs Clin North Am 1998
Sep;10(3):267-78
Care of the critically ill client at home.
McNeal GJ.
Keystone Mercy Health Plan, Philadelphia,
Pennsylvania, USA.
The high-tech homecare nurse is
operationalizing the trend to bring critical
care nursing and medical services directly
to the homecare environment. With the
continuing advancement in technologic
capability, the role of this newly emerging
critical care nurse clinician will grow in
scope of practice. As the health care
industry strives to create more cost-
effective solutions to the nation's burden of
health care delivery, the relocation of
complex medical interventions to the
homecare setting is one method of
effecting a seamless health care delivery
system, where quality of care is maintained
while costs are controlled.

Crit Care Nurs Clin North Am 1998
Sep;10(3):339-46
Pediatric considerations in homecare.
Petit de Mange EA.
Department of Nursing, West Chester
University, Pennsylvania, USA.
epetitdemange@wcupa.edu
"If I had known beforehand how difficult,
demanding, time consuming, and
exhausting it would be--having my child
home on a ventilator--I would never have
agreed to bring her home" (personal
communication with a parent, 1994). This
mother's statement strikes at the heart of
pediatric high-tech homecare. Parents
assume caregiver roles that professional
health providers have taken years to
develop. Nurses, as strangers, intrude into
intimate family relationships that have
cultivated over years. Pioneering agencies
attempt to fill a gap in pediatric care using
guidelines that have been entrenched in the
medical and economic models for years.
The multiple dimensions of high-tech
pediatric homecare require more than
provision of technical nursing services. In
homecare, nurses are challenged by
cultural differences, language barriers, loss

of control, family dynamics, practicing in
unfamiliar environments, and new
technology. To ensure quality nursing care,
all professional dimensions need to be
considered to be of equal importance.

Crit Care Nurs Q 1996 Feb;18(4):16-25
The challenge of handling chemotherapy in
the intensive care unit.
Alfafara AA, Hedges L.
Newer, more intensive cancer treatments
and even some standard treatments in
critically ill cancer patients mandate
provision of care in the intensive care unit
(ICU). Traditionally, the ICU nurse has not
had specialized training in the preparation
or administration of chemotherapeutic
agents. This article discusses educational
needs and specific information related to
safe handling of chemotherapy
administration.

Crit Care Nurs Q 1996 May;19(1):65-72
Caring for the lesbian, gay, or bisexual
patient: issues for critical care nurses.
Eliason MJ.
Critical care nurses have a moral obligation
to provide quality care for all of their
patients. Many nurses lack information
about lesbian, gay, and bisexual patient
issues or feel uncomfortable working with
such clients. This article explores some of
the stereotypes that create negative
attitudes about lesbian, gay, and bisexual
people and offers suggestions for critical
care nurses who wish to become better
educated about these clients.

Crit Care Nurs Q 1997 Aug;20(2):1-5
Critical care in Nicaragua.
Simko LC.
Duquesne University, School of Nursing,
Clinical Nurse II, Western Pennsylvania
Hospital Pittsburgh, USA.
Critical care nursing in Nicaragua is vastly
different than critical care practiced in the
United States. The current status of critical
care nursing in Nicaragua is challenging at
best. Medical personnel do not have access
to arterial blood gases, blood cultures, and
capillary blood glucose monitoring. The
strengths and challenges present in
Nicaraguan critical care has made the

nursing staff rely on keen and astute nursing assessment of their patients. Due to the lack of technology in Nicaragua, creativity and improvising are a must in caring for a critically ill patient. However, the concerns and issues facing the nurses in Nicaragua are very similar to those experienced by critical care nurses in the United States. Critical care nursing in Nicaragua is indeed true nursing at its finest.

Crit Care Nurs Q 1997 Aug;20(2):22-7
Application of pulse oximetry and the oxyhemoglobin dissociation curve in respiratory management.
Goodfellow LM.
Duquesne University School of Nursing, University of Pittsburgh School of Nursing, Pennsylvania, USA.
Teaching the principles of respiratory management in a developing Spanish-speaking country presents many challenges. It is futile, for example, to present content on blood gas analysis when the equipment to analyze blood gases is not available. However, pulse oximetry in available in many of these countries and can be used to manage the patient's oxygen flow rates or ventilator changes. This article explores the value of the oxyhemoglobin dissociation curve in this context and also reinforces the basic principles of pulse oximetry in respiratory management for nurses in the United States and abroad.

Crit Care Nurs Q 1999 May;22(1):1-7
The suspiciousness factor: critical care nursing and forensics.
Winfrey ME, Smith AR.
Department of Adult and Gerontological Nursing, College of Nursing, University of Massachusetts, Boston, USA.
This conceptual article provides a guide for understanding the place of forensic nursing within the discipline of nursing. Ways of knowing in nursing and expert nursing practice are described to identify the role of intuition in nursing practice. The relationship between suspicion and intuition is explored. Strategies for developing forensic nursing expertise and

increasing suspicion are described. Suspicion (intuition) is presented as a rapid, acquired, patient oriented perception that leads to decisive action.

Crit Care Nurse 1997 Apr;17(2):64-70
Managing a shift effectively: the role of the charge nurse.
Osguthorpe SG.
Nursing Service for Medicine and Surgery, Salt Lake City Veterans Affairs Medical Center, Utah, USA.

Crit Care Nurse 1998 Feb;18(1):40-51
Renal replacement therapy in critical care: implementation of a unit-based continuous venovenous hemodialysis program.
Giuliano KK, Pysznik EE.
Baystate Medical Center, Springfield, Mass., USA.
Implementing a program as complex as continuous venovenous hemodialysis without the involvement of nephrology nurses is a challenge. However, with proper planning, appropriate staff support, and the ability to make changes as implementation proceeds, a successful program can be developed. Our reward is that we are now able to offer a therapy that is important and potentially lifesaving to those critically ill patients with renal failure who are unable to tolerate intermittent hemodialysis.

Crit Care Nurse 1999 Dec;19(6):54-63
Continuous arteriovenous rewarming: a bedside technique.
Schulman CS, Pierce B.
Harborview Medical Center, Seattle, Wash., USA.

Crit Care Nurse 1999 Feb;19(1):34-44
Improving the care of cardiothoracic surgery patients through advanced nursing skills.
Zevola DR, Maier B.
Cardiothoracic Intensive Care Unit, Westchester Medical Center, Valhalla, NY, USA.
All the nurses in the cardiothoracic ICU are now certified in these advanced skills. The skills are reviewed with current staff members on a yearly basis during the

annual evaluation. During their orientation to the cardiothoracic ICU, new staff nurses are certified by using the original process of attending an in-service training program and demonstrating the skill 3 times. The quality management department reviews medical records daily to detect complications. In addition, we (DRZ and MB) conducted a quality assurance review in which we monitored 20 patients being extubated and having PA catheters removed by nurses. No complications were noted during either review. The institution has seen improvements in quality of care and earlier discharge from the hospital. With earlier removal of endotracheal tubes and PA catheters, patients are more comfortable and their rehabilitation can be advanced sooner. Comparison of the mean length of stay for patients undergoing coronary artery bypass graft in March 1995 with the mean length of stay for such patients in March 1998 showed a 50.6% decrease, from 14.94 days to 7.38 days. These advanced skills have provided an increased autonomy for the nurses and have benefited the patients undergoing cardiac surgery in our institution.

CRNA 2000 Feb;11(1):41-8
Patient safety and human error: the big picture.
Gunn IP.
For most of the past century, health care literature including many books written about health care and its quality have documented the problems of errors in health care delivery. That outcomes of care have differed significantly among hospitals has also inferred that perhaps the "best practices" or the appropriate resources may not have been used, although most of these study results have be adjusted for case mix. The Institute of Medicine's recent publication, "To Err is Human," represents their review of studies quantifying medical errors in health care and their recommendations for eliminating such errors to the extent possible. One should note that, while using the term "medical," it does not infer that all errors are made by physicians. It recommends shifting the focus of study from blaming the health providers to studying the "system" in which health care is provided, believing that most of the errors committed are not reckless but rather result from system variables. The Institute of Medicine's recommendations are broad and cover a variety of quality assurance mechanisms. It recommends mandatory reporting of these errors to a central agency via a state mechanism, with better and broader legislation to make peer review, for purposes of studying errors with a view toward making change in the system, privileged information, and not subject to subpoena. The American Medical Association and American Nurses Association, in their testimony before the US Senate Committee on Appropriations, Subcommittee on Labor, Health and Human Services, Education and Related Agencies, on December 13, 1999, support the recommendations in general with a few reservations.

Dermatol Nurs 1998 Jun;10(3):183-8
Handwashing in health care.
Mayone-Ziomek JM.
Arizona State University, Tempe, USA.
Noncompliance with handwashing is a significant problem in the health care setting. Numerous studies demonstrate that strategies can be implemented to improve compliance with handwashing. This information has relevance for all areas of nursing practice.

Dimens Crit Care Nurs 1997 May-Jun;16(3):152-62
A model for teaching critical thinking in the clinical setting.
Whiteside C.
As the scope of nursing practice changes, the ability of nurses to think critically and make appropriate clinical judgements becomes even more necessary. The author shares a model for teaching critical thinking and describes how it can be used to improve the critical thinking skills of critical care nurses.

Dimens Crit Care Nurs 1997 Nov-Dec;16(6):314-23; quiz 324
Recognizing the potential for violence in

the ICU.
Drury T.
Denver Health Medical Center, CO, USA.
Violence in health care institutions, specifically critical care units, throughout the country is increasing at an alarming rate. This problem is not confined to the urban areas but also encompasses rural regions. This article assists the nurse in identifying the potential for violence by patients, family, or visitors while they are in the critical care unit. The author describes strategies that have been successful in controlling violence in the ICU and suggests steps nurse educators and managers can take to reduce the risk of violence in their units. The article is followed by Education STATPack material that can be used by current subscribers for an inservice.

Drug Saf 2000 Apr;22(4):321-33
Drug-related problems in hospitalised patients.
van den Bemt PM, Egberts TC, de Jong-van den Berg LT, Brouwers JR.
Hospital Pharmacy Medisch Centrum Leeuwarden, De Tjongerschans Hospital, Heerenveen, The Netherlands.
bemtp@mcz-nw.znb.nl
Drug-related problems include medication errors (involving an error in the process of prescribing, dispensing, or administering a drug, whether there are adverse consequences or not) and adverse drug reactions (any response to a drug which is noxious and unintended, and which occurs at doses normally used in humans for prophylaxis, diagnosis or therapy of disease, or for the modification of physiological function). Furthermore, adverse drug events can be defined as an injury--whether or not causally-related to the use of a drug. Drug-related problems are relatively common in hospitalised patients and can result in patient morbidity and mortality, and increased costs. In order to get an overview of studies on drug-related problems in hospitalised patients, with specific attention to the incidence of drug-related problems and their costs, to the possibilities of prevention and to the effect of these interventions, we performed

a literature search. Incidences of medication errors reported in studies vary widely. The range of reported incidences of adverse drug reactions is even wider. These wide ranges can be largely explained by the different study methods and definitions used. Problems related to drug therapy may be averted by preventive interventions. Several possibilities for prevention exist, especially for the prevention of medication errors. Prescribing, transcription and interpretation errors can be reduced by using computerised physician order entry. Together with the use of automated dispensing systems and bar-code technology, this will aid in the reduction of both dispensing and administration errors. Education of nursing staff involved in the process of drug distribution is another important measure for preventing medication errors. Finally, the introduction of systems for the early detection of adverse drug reactions may help to reduce problems related to drug therapy. Identifying risk factors that contribute to the development of adverse drug reactions, may aid in the prevention of these reactions.

East Afr Med J 1996 Dec;73(12):830-1
Surgery and training in surgery in remote rural hospitals.
Steiner AK.
Addis Ababa University, Ethiopia.
Surgery is an important part of primary health care in remote rural areas of third world countries. It is essential that doctors and nurses who are working in rural hospitals are adequately trained in surgery. Special consideration should be given to the surgical pathology encountered in the rural tropical environment. Teaching should take place in the set-up of the rural hospital and should include anaesthesia, sterilisation and maintenance of equipment. A concept of teaching in surgery in peripheral hospitals is presented.

EDTNA ERCA J 1996 Jul-Sep;22(3):33-5
Trauma counselling: what is it and does it exist within the caring professions?
Beddoes P.

Southmead Hospital, Southmead Health Trust.

EDTNA ERCA J 1998 Apr-Jun;24(2):7-10
Prolonging access function and survival, the nurse's role.
Hayes J.
Oxford Renal Unit, Oxford Radcliffe Hospitals NHS Trust Renal Unit, Churchill Hospital, Headington, UK.
Vascular access is the lifeline of all patients undergoing HD. In a recent patient satisfaction survey, the area of vascular access and needling technique was highlighted as an area with the need for improvement, this is addressed in this paper by the formulation of: Individual access Vulnerability Score, an Access Care Plan and the implementation of a Staff cannulation training programme. Addressing these 3 areas of practice with a structured programme not only assists staff to develop and value patient access but ultimately provides a higher quality of service. Patient satisfaction, access complications, staff knowledge and clinical abilities can all be improved by the implementation of a more structured approach to developing and valuing vascular access.

EDTNA ERCA J 1998 Oct-Dec;24(4):11-4
Quality decision making in dialysis.
Nilsson LG, Anderberg C, Ipsen R, Persson E, Andersson G.
Gambro AB, Lund, Sweden.
A patient approaching the final stage of his renal disease is faced with many difficult questions. Should he opt for a transplant or start on dialysis? In the case of dialysis, can he manage his treatment at home or will he need to be cared for in a clinic? Should be choose peritoneal dialysis or haemodialysis? Is the freedom of being independent from a machine, given by CAPD, as valuable as the freedom of having days without treatment, given by HD? The issues are complex and do not have a given answer. To make the proper decisions about his treatment the patient needs extensive information and support from the caregivers. Likewise, the caregivers need to know the patient well in order to give appropriate advice. In this exchange of information, the renal nurse has a very important role. Some patients may need to be dialysed in a hospital but most can get an equally good or even better dialysis treatment in a less stressful environment. A high degree of self-care is preferred by people who value independence and freedom of movement. Self-care also improves the self-confidence and increases the chances of maintaining employment and a rich social life. Self-care could mean both PD and HD, sometimes with the assistance of a spouse or a nurse. But a certain degree of self-care can also be maintained in limited-care centres and satellites, where the presence of nursing staff gives the feeling of security. For everybody involved, not least the purchasers of health care, it is desirable to keep the patients out of the costly hospital environment for as long as possible.

Elder Care 1998 Dec-1999 Jan;10(6):18-20
Staying out.
Bloodworth C.
Queens Medical Centre, Nottingham.

Elder Care 1998 Oct-Nov;10(5):17-9
The construction of challenging behaviour.
Innes A, Jacques I.
Bradford Dementia Group, Anchor Trust, Altrincham.

Emerg Med Clin North Am 1991 Nov;9(4):881-4
Quality assurance for the radiology-emergency interface.
Bauman TW, Bauman DH.
Bauman Radiologists, Inc., Allison Park, Pennsylvania.
Quality assurance does not have to be a dirty word. Developing indicators, identifying trends, taking action, and reassessing the results can significantly benefit the technical and nursing staff, emergency physicians, radiologists, and, especially, the patients.

Emerg Nurse 1998 Apr;6(1):12-6
Major incident planning particularly those including chemicals.

Wheeler H.
Chemical Incident Response Service,
Medical Toxicology Unit, Guys' and St
Thomas' Hospital Trust, London.
A chemical incident can happen anytime,
anywhere and is often complex in nature.
Henrietta Wheeler advises on the necessary
precautions staff must take to avoid the
risk of poisoning and contamination to
both staff and casualties.

Emerg Nurse 1998 Jun;6(3):22-7
Critical incident stress management
strategies.
Cudmore J.
Great Ormond Street Hospital for Sick
Children.

Emerg Nurse 1998 Oct;6(6):25-8
Principles of universal precautions.
Perry C, Barnett J.
United Bristol Healthcare NHS Trust.

Emerg Nurse 1999 Apr;7(1):12-6
Interpersonal approaches to managing
violence and aggression.
Morcombe J.
A&E Department, Children's Hospital,
Sheffield.

Emerg Nurse 1999 Feb;6(9):24-7
Why A&E nurses feel inadequate in
managing patients who deliberately self
harm?
Perego M.
Bristol Royal Infirmary.

Enferm Intensiva 1998 Oct-Dec;9(4):160-8
[Cardiopulmonary resuscitation in
pregnant women: peculiarities]
[Article in Spanish]
Grau Gandia S, Martinez Ramon MA.
Servicio de Urgencias Obstetrico-
Ginecologicas del Hospital Virgen del
Castillo Yecla, Murcia.
This review main purpose is to show
nursing the present knowledge about
cardiopulmonary resuscitation (CPR) in
pregnant women because of the scarce
information published by Spanish Nursing
Publications. The bibliographical research
was made using both the Medline (from
January 1982 to March 1998) and Index de

Enfermeria databases. There, we can find
32 references from which only 23 were
selected (all of them belong to the Medline
database) in spite of 3 chapters that had
already been selected from other different
books. Although maternal cardiac arrest
rarely happens during pregnancy, it is very
important for sanitary staff to be
familiarized with the specifics thecnics and
equipment (ultrasound and
cardiotocograph monitoring). This review
describes the physiological changes that
take place during pregnancy and have an
incidence into CPR. The article also
includes the conclusions about the checked
papers and the peculiarities that have to be
taken into account in each CPR, such as
the fetal viability evaluation, right CPR
position, airway and breathing,
desfibrillation, external cardiac
compression and use of pharmacologic
therapy and intravenous fluids. Moreover,
there is a special mention of the
perimortem cesarean delivery features:
antecedents, foetus-maternals
consequences and managements, due to the
fact that this surgical operation should be
included inside the CPR protocols of the
pregnant.

Gastroenterol Nurs 1998 Sep-Oct;21(5):207-9
The benefits of patient education.
Abbott SA.
St. Paul Endoscopy Center, MN 55102,
USA.
In this article, the role of the nurse in
patient education is described, as well as
the benefits of patient education, such as
improved quality of care, improved patient
satisfaction, increased compliance,
improved staff satisfaction, and effective
use of resources. Strategies for effective
patient teaching also are presented.

Geriatr Nurs 1996 Mar-Apr;17(2):81-5
A controlled evaluation of a lifts and
transfer educational program for nurses.
Gray J, Cass J, Harper DW, O'Hara PA.
Publication Types: Clinical Trial,
Randomized Controlled Trial Review,
Review, Tutorial

Geriatr Nurs 1997 May-Jun;18(3):115-8
  Identification and assistance for chemically
  dependent nurses working in long-term
  care.
  Shewey HM.
  Kansas Department of Health and
  Environment, Topeka, USA.
  The purpose of this manuscript is to
  examine impaired nurses' practice, to
  identify causes, signs, and symptoms of
  problems, and to identify interventions for
  chemically dependent nurses employed in
  long-term care. The long-term care nurse
  manager has a moral, ethical, and legal
  responsibility to assist the chemically
  dependent nurse and to protect the resident
  and the facility. Education of nurse
  managers is essential to provide for
  intervention and treatment for the
  chemically dependent nurse. Assisting the
  nurse to accept treatment and return to
  practice benefits the individuals, the
  facility, and the profession. This
  manuscript describes step-by-step
  interventions for identification, treatment,
  and return to work for chemically
  dependent nurses.

Geriatr Nurs 1999 Jan-Feb;20(1):14-7
  Challenges for Australian nursing in the
  International Year of Older Persons.
  Nay R, Garratt S, Koch S.
  School of Nursing, La Trobe University,
  Melbourne, Australia.
  Some of the major issues challenging
  gerontic nursing in Australia are addressed
  in this article. The broad context of change
  that has been introduced by successive
  Australian governments is presented
  briefly. The problems of attracting and
  keeping qualified nurses in aged care
  exacerbated by a trend toward employers
  actively seeking to replace qualified nurses
  with unregulated staff are discussed.
  Education and work practice changes are
  proposed as minimum responses required
  from nursing if the profession is to remain
  relevant and central to aged care into the
  21st century.

Geriatr Nurs 1999 Nov-Dec;20(6):309-13
  Care of the morbidly obese patient in a
  long-term care facility.
  Rotkoff N.
  Treetops Nursing Home, Mohegan Lake,
  N.Y., USA.
  Morbidly obese patients in a long-term
  care (LTC) facility have special physical
  and emotional needs that must be
  considered when planning care. Special
  attention to the skin, vital sign monitoring,
  and rehabilitative care are among the
  interventions that must be integrated into
  the otherwise standard care of the morbidly
  obese patient. A case study is used to
  illustrate the challenges and special needs
  of such patients in an LTC facility in New
  York state. Morbidly obese people
  (nonambulatory people who are obese)
  frequently are unable to perform self-care.
  The care of the morbidly obese adult who
  resides in an LTC or postacute care
  facility, in particular, offers unique
  challenges to nursing staff.

Health Care Women Int 1999 Mar-
  Apr;20(2):209-19
  Nursing's role in racism and African
  American women's health.
  Eliason MJ.
  College of Nursing, University of Iowa,
  Iowa City 52242, USA. mickey-
  eliason@uiowa.edu
  African American women's health has been
  neglected in the nursing and other health
  care literature, in spite of evidence that
  they are among the most vulnerable
  populations in the United States today. In
  this article, I highlight the health disparities
  between African American and European
  American women, discuss possible reasons
  for the disparities, and propose that nursing
  as a profession has been complicit in
  perpetuating the racism of health care and
  society. Although the focus is on nursing
  research and practice, it is likely that other
  health care disciplines perpetuate racism in
  similar ways.

Heart Lung 1998 Nov-Dec;27(6):355-9
  Comment in: Heart Lung. 1999 May-
  Jun;28(3):226
  A challenge for clinical nurses: a new
  nursing role.
  Balogh D, Berry A.
  Intensive Care Unit, Nepean Hospital,

Penrith, New South Wales, Australia. As a result of difficulties in attracting resident medical officers (RMOs) to the outer western suburbs of Sydney, the intensive care unit at Nepean Hospital created a new nursing position in 1992 called the clinical assistant (CA). This position was trialed and, after a successful period in the intensive care unit, it was expanded to the surgical, pediatric, and mental health divisions. The generic job description of the CA is comprehensive and includes advanced clinical, educational, research, and managerial components. There are a number of variations within the areas of practice. For example, within the clinical component, the intensive care CA is expected to be able to insert central venous and arterial catheters, whereas the mental health CA adopts a full caseload and is responsible for patient assessment and management. A working party was established in 1995 and comprised previous and current CAs, an education manager, a senior nursing administrator, and representatives from personnel and the New South Wales Nursing Association (nursing union). The working party conducted an extensive evaluation of this new nursing role, and the recommendations that followed received a positive response from the hospital management.

Home Healthc Nurse 1996 Oct;14(10):803-12
Productivity in home healthcare: Part II: Maintaining and improving nurse performance.
Benefield LE.
Harris College of Nursing, Texas Christian University, Fort Worth, USA.

Home Healthc Nurse 1996 Sep;14(9):698-706
Productivity in home healthcare: part I: assessing nurse effectiveness and efficiency.
Benefield LE.
Herein described is a profile of the specific knowledge and abilities of the productive home care RN that nurse managers can use in maintaining and developing an RN staff that is efficient and effective. This article describes the profile and shows how it can be used in the hiring process, during orientation, and on a day-to-day basis to manage and improve the productivity of current staff members.

Hosp Health Serv Adm 1994 Spring;39(1):47-62
Capitalizing on the recession's effect on hospital RN shortages.
Buerhaus PI.
Harvard School of Public Health, Department of Health Policy and Management, Boston, MA 02115.
The recent economic recession and slow-paced recovery have contributed to dampening out the shortage of hospital-employed registered nurses (RNs), a shortage that has persisted since the mid-1980s. While national unemployment rates remain relatively high and continue to exert economic pressure on RNs to maintain high levels of employment activity, hospital and nurse executives now have an opportunity to make strategic investments in the organizational infrastructure supporting nursing because once the economy rebounds, RN shortages could easily resurface.

Image J Nurs Sch 1998;30(4):323-7
Use of immigration policy to manage nursing shortages.
Glaessel-Brown EE.
Journeylines, Boston, MA 02130, USA.
egblines@world.std.com
PURPOSE: To examine long-term implications of using temporary, nonimmigrant nurse programs to manage fluctuations in the demand for registered nurses.
ORGANIZING FRAMEWORK: This discussion is located in the full context of migration--reviewing theories and concepts of labor migration--referring to experience with guest-worker programs worldwide, outlining recent nursing shortages in the United States, describing the Immigration Nursing Relief Act (INRA), and raising questions for nurses in the United States and in the global marketplace.
SOURCES: Review of scholarly literature on international migration, existing studies on nurse migration to the United States,

and original research, conducted between 1992 and 1994, for the Immigration Nursing Relief Advisory Committee (INRAC) Report.

METHODS: Policy analysis of theories, concepts, and perspectives related to nurse migration.

FINDINGS: In the United States, highly skilled foreign nurses tend to complement rather than displace local labor. Yet recruiting foreign-educated nurses for entry-level jobs perpetuates patterns of dependency in the sending country and delays creative solutions to staff development in the host country. Nonimmigrant status creates a vulnerable workforce. There may be a disparity between the ideal of nurse migration as collaborative exchange and the reality of institutionalized occupational migration networks.

CONCLUSIONS: While foreign nurse recruitment might solve short-term needs, repetitive temporary nurse migration programs create long-term consequences that are not in the best interests of the profession. The absence of consistent policy creates an opportunity for nursing to take an active role in developing the rules and direction of future nurse migration.

Image J Nurs Sch 1999;31(4):399-401
Nursing and the health system in Brazil.
Villa TC, Assis MM, Mishima SM, Pereira MJ, de Almeida MC, Palha PF, Pinto IC.
University of Sao Paulo, Ribeirao Preto College of Nursing, WHO Collaborating Centre for Nursing Research Development. tite@glete.eerp.usp.br
The purpose of this article is to describe nursing in the Brazilian health system and to analyze the characteristics of nursing personnel in Brazil. This description includes types of health institutions, services rendered, and the distribution of nursing personnel by professional categories in 1956, 1982, and 1995. Discussion of the challenges facing Brazilian nurses is presented using data from the Brazilian Institute of Geography and Statistics (IBGE), Federal Nursing Board (COFEn), Regional Nursing Board (COREn), and the Brazilian Nursing Association (ABEn). An increase in the number of outpatient units and in diagnostic and therapeutic examinations has led to an increased the demand for nurses. Public health nurses participate in planning, management, sanitary education, health promotion, and supervision of nursing care provided by nursing technicians, assistants, and other helpers.

Image J Nurs Sch 1999;31(4):399-401
Nursing and the health system in Brazil.
Villa TC, Assis MM, Mishima SM, Pereira MJ, de Almeida MC, Palha PF, Pinto IC.
University of Sao Paulo, Ribeirao Preto College of Nursing, WHO Collaborating Centre for Nursing Research Development. tite@glete.eerp.usp.br
The purpose of this article is to describe nursing in the Brazilian health system and to analyze the characteristics of nursing personnel in Brazil. This description includes types of health institutions, services rendered, and the distribution of nursing personnel by professional categories in 1956, 1982, and 1995. Discussion of the challenges facing Brazilian nurses is presented using data from the Brazilian Institute of Geography and Statistics (IBGE), Federal Nursing Board (COFEn), Regional Nursing Board (COREn), and the Brazilian Nursing Association (ABEn). An increase in the number of outpatient units and in diagnostic and therapeutic examinations has led to an increased the demand for nurses. Public health nurses participate in planning, management, sanitary education, health promotion, and supervision of nursing care provided by nursing technicians, assistants, and other helpers.

Imprint 1998 Apr-May;45(3):31-4
Moments of courage reconciling the real and ideal in the clinical practicum.
Savage TA, Bosek MS.
College of Nursing, University of Illinois, Chicago, USA.

Imprint 1998 Apr-May;45(3):37-9
Maintaining patient confidentiality in today's health care environment.

Allen K.

Imprint 1998 Apr-May;45(3):43-5
Nursing and ethical issues.
Ramsey GC.
New York University, School of
Education, Division of Nursing, USA.

Int J Nurs Pract 1996 Sep;2(3):122-8
The triage role in emergency nursing:
development of an educational programme.
McNally S.
University of Western Sydney Nepean,
New South Wales, Australia.
This study explores the professional and
educational development of emergency
nurses and their beliefs regarding the
appropriate content for a triage educational
programme. A descriptive survey was
conducted of emergency nurses employed
by randomly selected teaching and non-
teaching hospitals. Data analysis showed
that emergency nurses used various
methods to prepare and maintain their
triage expertise. The survey found that the
best method to prepare the novice
emergency nurse for the triage role was to
use a combination of a triage educational
programme and clinical experience.
Respondents indicated great interest in
enrolling in an educational programme
and, as a result of this survey, a
comprehensive triage educational
programme has been developed.
Publication Types: Review; Review
Literature

Int J Nurs Pract 1996 Sep;2(3):142-8
The need to develop nursing practice
through innovation and practice change.
Wright SG.
European Nursing Development Agency,
United Kingdom.
This paper examines some of the strategies
that can be used to produce change in
nursing. These strategies range from the
power-coercive through rational-empirical
to the normative-re-educative. Strategies
that promote a 'bottom-up' approach are
advocated for clinical nursing and some of
the principal factors towards success, such
as team building, the presence of a clinical
leader and planning are indicated. The

paper will also expand on what needs to be
changed in nursing, and what the purpose
of such changes are. It is argued that
externally focused efforts of change, such
as the organization of care or new practices
are only part of the picture. The journey of
change also requires an inner exploration
of who we are and what are we seeking to
achieve in nursing.

Int J Nurs Pract 2000 Feb;6(1):2-6
Luck: what the nurse should know about it
and how it affects nursing situations.
Shearer R, Davidhizar R.
Bethel College, Mishawaka, Indiana, USA.
Luck permeates every aspect of human
behaviour. Thus, luck is an aspect of
nursing care and client belief of which the
nurse should be aware. Beliefs about luck
will influence client compliance with
recommendations for actions as well as
influence actions the client selects in
relation to health. Beliefs about luck will
also influence actions the nurse may take
when responding to clients.

Int J Nurs Stud 1996 Feb;33(1):67-75
The role of the nurse in patient-focused
care: models of competence and
implications for education and training.
Burchell H, Jenner EA.
School of Humanities and Education,
University of Hertfordshire, Hatfield, UK.
This article explores implications of
Patient-Focused Care (PFC) for the
education and training of nurses. It does so
by examining various models of
competence and their strengths and
limitations as bases for developing training
programmes. It cautions against attempting
to transpose an approach to training based
on the U.S.A. model of PFC without
modification, given the differing nursing
roles in the U.K. PFC setting. It argues for
a broad-based definition of competence
rather than a narrower focus on training in
specific skills alone.
Publication Types: Review; Review
Literature

Int J Palliat Nurs 2000 Feb;6(2):58-65
Issues in effective pain control. 1:
Assessment and education.

Davies J, McVicar A.
School of Health Care Practice, Anglia
Polytechnic University, Chelmsford, UK.
Pain is a complex phenomenon to which an
individual's response is determined by the
interactions of physical, psychological,
cultural and social factors (Melzack and
Wall, 1988; Woodward, 1995; Horn and
Munafo, 1997). It cannot be measured, and
self-assessment by patients is increasingly
recognized as the most accurate means of
evaluating their pain. However, research
indicates that even self-assessment remains
problematic because nurses frequently
either do not use pain tools effectively, or
do not always accept the self-assessment.
Reasons for this seem to be rooted in the
attitudes and beliefs of nurses, and
inadequate communication. The latter
problem could be improved by more
effective use of pain tools, but attitudinal
problems are more difficult to address once
the barriers have become established. This
article suggests that the most effective way
to prevent such barriers arising is to ensure
that nurses receive a focused, substantive
input on pain assessment and pain control
within their preregistration studies.
Referring to proposals put forward several
years ago by the Royal College of Nursing
(Davis and Seers, 1991), the authors
suggest that the process should begin very
early in preregistration studies, preferably
within the first 6 months, and involve
teaching and learning strategies that
encourage personal exploration and so are
conducive to personal growth and
development. In this way, postregistration
studies could realistically focus on
specialist aspects of pain care more
appropriate to 'continuing education'.

Int J Psychiatr Nurs Res 2000 Jun;6(1):650-6
Real time training for mental health staff
working in an in-patient setting.
Hardcastle M.
BAHardcastle@Compuserve.com
Concerns around acute in-patient mental
health care including staff training are
becoming increasingly prominent
(Sainsbury, 1998; Sainsbury 1997). A
training solution is proposed in this paper,

which aims to deliver content derived from
evidence based practice actually within the
practitioner's own clinical workplace
during their working hours. The benefits of
this approach are discussed together with
examples of content and methods for
evaluating learning outcomes.

Intensive Crit Care Nurs 1996 Aug;12(4):193-9
Staffing intensive care units: a
consideration of contemporary issues.
Endacott R.
Intensive care nurses are an expensive and
scarce resource. The internal market within
the National Health Service requires
greater scrutiny of expenditure in all areas,
not least staffing. Inevitably questions are
raised regarding the evidence to justify the
nurse:patient ratios in specialist areas such
as intensive care. This paper addresses
some of the issues surrounding staffing in
intensive care and discusses the impact of
changes in medical practice on the nursing
role. The nurse:patient ratio is lower in the
USA, therefore a brief comparison between
the two countries is provided in order to
inform discussion and debate. The
importance of these issues for all intensive
care nurses is emphasised, together with a
plea for a substantive study to provide
evidence of nursing work and inform
future decision-making by the purchasers
and providers of intensive care services.

Intensive Crit Care Nurs 1997 Aug;13(4):230-7
Aspects of pulmonary artery
catheterization in critical care.
Storey LJ.
Coronary Care Unit, Hull Royal Infirmary,
East Yorkshire, UK.
The concept of floating a balloon-tipped
catheter into the pulmonary artery was first
described in 1970 by Swan et al. Since
then, many issues have surrounded the use
of these catheters. Of particular concern for
many physicians was the incidence of
complications associated with use of the
catheters. A group of clinicians have
endeavoured to show the usefulness of the
pulmonary artery catheter (PAC), but
showing significant improvement to patient
outcome has proved difficult. Physicians

and nurses have demonstrated poor knowledge and skills associated with use of the catheter which must be overcome before conclusive benefits of the catheter can be demonstrated. Training nurses to use a PAC correctly has been highlighted in reducing the number of technical problems associated with the catheter, which in turn improves the accuracy of haemodynamic data obtained. Unfortunately, training programmes are few and far between, and this is an issue that must be addressed by critical care nurse managers. In this review of the literature regarding PACs and their use in the care of the critically ill patients, the role of the nurse is discussed with recommendations for practice.

Intensive Crit Care Nurs 1997 Jun;13(3):151-5
Nursing perspectives for intensive care.
Woodrow P.
Middlesex University, Whittington Education Centre, London, UK.
Within health care, market forces increasingly determine what services have economic value. For nursing to survive this economic onslaught, nurses must clarify their values and roles. While nurses working in intensive care develop useful technical skills and normally work within a constructive multi-disciplinary team framework, they have a potentially unique contribution to care, focusing on the patient as a whole person rather than intervening to solve a problem. The need for both physiological and psychological care creates a need for holistic values, best achieved through humanistic perspectives. Humanistic nursing places patients as people at the centre of nursing care, as illustrated by the limitations of reality orientation compared with the potentials of validation therapy. Intensive care nurses asserting and developing such patient-centred roles offer a valuable way forward for nursing to develop into the 21st century.

Intensive Crit Care Nurs 1997 Jun;13(3):167-9
Ethical decision-making in intensive care: are nurses suitable patient advocates?

Norrie P.
Department of Health and Continuing Professional Studies, De Montfort University, Leicester, UK.
According to the United Kingdom Central Council for Nursing, Midwifery and Health Visiting (UKCC) code of conduct (1992), nurses in Britain are expected to act as patient advocates. An advocate is someone who 'pleads for another' (Concise Oxford Dictionary 1982). However, it has been shown that advocacy is a complex issue and it is debatable as to whether or not it is a legitimate attribute of the role of the nurse (Gates 1995). Mallik (1997) also finds that advocacy can be a risky career option. Professional codes of conduct spell out duties, but do not give moral guidance. Phrases such as 'promote and safeguard the well-being of the patient' (UKCC 1992) are used, but although undoubtedly well-intentioned, this is platitudinous and these codes commonly shed little light on how to define an action that is to the patient's benefit or detriment. It is tempting to suggest that they are used as a drunken man uses a street lamp; more for support than illumination. Castledine (1981) identified a number of factors that would make a nurse an inappropriate advocate and these will be discussed within the context of intensive care units (ICUs).

Intensive Crit Care Nurs 1998 Aug;14(4):203-7
Family nursing in intensive care. Part two: The needs of a family with a member in intensive care.
Robb YA.
Glasgow Caledonian University, UK.
It was demonstrated in Part one that the family is a justifiable concern to nurses in intensive care and that family-focused care is appropriate in such an area. If this approach to care is to be considered, it is necessary to identify the needs of families when they have a member in an intensive care unit. This is a well-researched area and some of the relevant literature is discussed within this paper. Before this literature is addressed, an attempt is made to define the concept of need. The methodologies used in the identification of family needs could be adapted to explore

whether or not the needs of the families of patients in a particular intensive care unit are being met. This paper suggests that if it was shown that the meeting of family needs was an area of care which could be improved upon, then a family-centred approach to care would be a reasonable option. If however, it is shown that families already perceived their needs as being met, then changing the system of care to a more formal family nursing approach would seem to be unnecessary.

Intensive Crit Care Nurs 1998 Dec;14(6):283-7
Cardiac and circulatory assessment in intensive care units.
McGrath A, Cox CL.
Department of Adult Nursing, City University St Bartholomew School of Nursing and Midwifery, Whitechapel, London, UK.
As healthcare delivery changes in critical care, nursing continues to evolve and develop. Nursing skills are expanding to incorporate skills once seen as the remit of the medical profession. Nurses are now equipping themselves with the skills and knowledge that can enhance the care they provide to their patients. Assessment of patients is a major role in nursing and, by expanding assessment skills, nurses can ensure that patients receive the care most appropriate to their needs. Nurses in critical care settings are well placed to carry out a more detailed assessment, which can help to focus nursing care. This article describes the step-by-step process of undertaking a full and comprehensive cardiac and circulatory assessment in a clinical setting. It identifies many of the problems that patients may have and the signs that the nurse may note whilst undertaking the assessment.

Intensive Crit Care Nurs 1998 Dec;14(6):288-93
Should relatives of patients with cardiac arrest be invited to be present during cardiopulmonary resuscitation?
Offord RJ.
Intensive Care Unit, Gloucestershire Royal Hospital NHS Trust, Gloucester, UK.
Witnessing the attempted resuscitation of a loved one is likely to be traumatic and distressing. However, because the majority of patients requiring cardiopulmonary resuscitation (CPR) die, this raises the question, within the hospital environment, of whether relatives should be invited to be present. There is a distinct lack of nursing research available on this subject, particularly with regard to the possible long-term effects on relatives. Much of the information is anecdotal and focuses on the positive aspects of this practice. With particular reference to the intensive care unit (ICU), the discussion in this paper includes not only family presence during CPR from the perspective of the patient, relatives and healthcare professionals, but also the potential legal implications. Recommendations for nursing practice are offered.

Intensive Crit Care Nurs 1999 Aug;15(4):204-9
Critical analysis of access to and availability of intensive care.
Southgate HM.
Faculty of Health, South Bank University, London, UK.
In intensive care, there appears to be an ever-increasing demand for resources and it is widely recognized that there is often a shortage of vacant beds available, compounded by an inadequate level of appropriately qualified nursing staff. Either of these deficiencies may lead to delayed or even refused admission for a patient who is critically ill. This review of the literature contains examination of the access and availability of intensive care facilities within the National Health Service and discussion of the problems that arise in gaining admission to such facilities. Being refused admission to the local intensive care unit may have important implications for a critically ill patient, resulting in transfer to another hospital, perhaps many miles away, or inadequate treatment and care in a general ward. These issues are also examined and strategies for action are proposed.
Publication Types: Review; Review Literature

Isr J Med Sci 1996 Sep;32(9):705-10
The clinical learning environment.
Rotem A, Bloomfield L, Southon G.
School of Medical Education, University
of New South Wales, Sydney, Australia.
This paper presents a brief review of the
attributes of effective learning
environments in clinical settings. Recent
studies articulate the perceived importance
of social and organizational factors as
determinants of learning. Differences are
evident among hospitals and among
departments within hospitals with regard to
the quality of the learning environment
they offer. These differences are reflected
in the orientation towards teaching and
learning, the level of autonomy, variety
and workload, and the quality of
supervision and social support. Differences
are also evident in the type and quality of
opportunities for practice of important
skills and in the availability of educational
resources. These factors are perceived as
major determinants of the effectiveness of
learning in clinical settings. The
implications for clinical teachers and
administrators are discussed. The authors
argue that emphasis should be given to the
creation of supportive and well-organized
learning environments in clinical settings.
This may require a great emphasis on the
role of clinical teachers as designers of
opportunities for learning and managers of
learning resources.

J Adv Nurs 1992 Jan;17(1):113-20
The role of the paid non-professional
nursing helper: a review of the literature.
Dewar BJ, Clark JM.
Department of Nursing Studies, King's
College, University of London, England.
This paper presents an overview of
research into the role of paid non-
professional nursing helpers. This term
refers to auxiliaries, ward clerks,
healthcare assistants and support workers.
The focus of the review is on work carried
out on attitudes of qualified staff to the role
of the helper, role descriptions and the role
of the helper in different organizational
modes of work. Some of the research
reviewed in relation to the role description
and attitudes to the helper date back to

1978. However, the emphasis of the paper
is on research published in the past 3 years.
The research is reviewed against the
background of two theoretical frameworks,
both of which are perceived to be useful in
analysing the division of labour between
the nurse, the patient and the helper.
Publication Types: Review; Review
Literature

J Adv Nurs 1995 Feb;21(2):371-7
Determinants of changes in nurses'
behaviour after continuing education: a
literature review.
Francke AL, Garssen B, Huijer Abu-Saad
H.
Helen Dowling Institute for
Biopsychosocial Medicine, Rotterdam, The
Netherlands.
Nursing continuing-education programmes
may differ in the extent to which they
affect nursing practice. Differences may be
explained by characteristics of the
participants' background, the programme
itself, teacher(s), relationship between
participants, relationship between
participants and teacher(s), physical
environment during the programme,
participants' social system, knowledge,
skills and attitudes, and intention to
change. In this literature review, a model is
presented which integrates these variables
and which may be used to explain why
continuing-education programmes have no,
little or considerable effect. On the basis of
current scientific knowledge, colleagues'
and superiors' support emerges as the most
important determinant of behavioural
changes in nursing practice.

J Adv Nurs 1996 Jan;23(1):32-8
The use of different research
methodologies to evaluate the effectiveness
of programmes to improve the care of
patients in postoperative pain.
Allcock N.
Department of Nursing and Midwifery
Studies, University of Nottingham,
Medical School, Queen's Medical Centre,
England.
Much research has supported the
conclusion of the report from The Royal
College of Surgeons and College of

Anaesthetists (1990), London, England, that the relief of postoperative pain is in many cases unsatisfactory and calls for more research on the effectiveness of educational programmes. A prime aim of nursing research is to influence and to improve practice. In relation to postoperative pain Sofaer's (1985) study was an example of the use of a quasi-experimental approach to improve postoperative pain relief through nurse education. Sofaer suggests that although positive effects were demonstrated they may not have been sustained in the long term. Further, Sofaer suggests that action research may have produced a more sustainable change. This paper critically discusses the use of these two research methods in relation to this problem.

J Adv Nurs 1996 Jul;24(1):104-7
Preceptorship: a review of the literature.
Bain L.
Royal Hallamshire Hospital, Sheffield, England.
Preceptorship is an important part of the United Kingdom Central Council for Nursing's (UKCC) post-registration and practice recommendations. Therefore, there is a great need for educationalists and clinical practitioners to explore the issues surrounding preceptorship and come to informed decisions on how they intend to implement preceptor programmes. There is a need to identify existing knowledge and its application to practice based on the commonly occurring themes within the theoretical and empirical literature. This paper reviews the current literature addressing these themes of role definition, preceptor selection, preceptorship programmes, the preceptorship experience and the limitations of preceptorship in clinical practice.

J Adv Nurs 1996 Jun;23(6):1238-46
Work-related back pain in nurses.
Hignett S.
Nottingham City Hospital, England.
This summary draws together the findings form over 80 studies published over three decades. The studies reviewed are categorized into three groups: (a)

epidemiological; (b) 'testing out'; and (c) exploratory. There has been agreement on a number of points, in particular that nursing is among the high risk occupations with respect to low back problems, with a point prevalence of approximately 17%, an annual (period) prevalence of 40-50% and a lifetime prevalence of 35-80%. When considering the contributory factors there is some divergence, but one of the popular notions is generally proven, that more frequent patient handling appears to correlate with increased incidence of low back pain. However, the traditional approach of training in lifting and handling techniques alone has been shown to be of little, or no, long-term benefit and the value of ergonomics remains to be seen. Much work has also been done by taking aspects of nursing work into the laboratory, using experimental studies which have mostly focused on specific sub-tasks (of the generic task of patient handling), looking at specific transfers and procedures (e.g. bed to chair) or transfer techniques ('stoop versus squat'). Although a level of quantification can be made about the different techniques, it is questionable whether this is of any practical use, especially when considering the wide variation of loads encountered during manual handling of patients. The limitations of using quantitative methodologies is revealed in the very small number of exploratory studies. All of the studies cited in this review used methodologies based in the positivist paradigm. There does not appear to be any published work using participative or interview methods to obtain qualitative data which might identify contributory factors in the onset of occupational low back pain in nursing staff.

J Adv Nurs 1996 Mar;23(3):430-40
From research to practice: one organizational model for promoting research-based practice.
Kitson A, Ahmed LB, Harvey G, Seers K, Thompson DR.
National Institute for Nursing, Radcliffe Infirmary, Oxford, England.
This paper describes a framework used by

the National Institute for Nursing in Oxford to integrate research, development and practice. With the increasing attention given to the topic of how research findings are implemented into clinical practice, it was felt important to share the challenges that have arisen in attempting to combine traditional research activities with more practice-based development work. The emerging conceptual framework, structures and functions are described, highlighting the variety of partnerships to be established in order to achieve the goal of integrating research into practice. While the underpinning principles of the framework-generating knowledge, implementing research into practice and evaluating the effectiveness of programmes-are not new, it is the way they have been combined within an organizational structure that could be helpful to others considering such a strategy. Both the strengths and weaknesses of the framework are discussed, a number of conclusions drawn as to its robustness and consideration given to its replication.
Publication Types: Review; Review Literature

J Adv Nurs 1996 Mar;23(3):471-8
The organization of clinical supervision within the nursing profession: a review of the literature.
Fowler J.
School of Health and Community Studies, De Montfort University, Leicester, England.
There is a considerable amount of literature available on the subject of supervision within the nursing profession. However, there appears to be little structure regarding how this subject is organized within the professional literature. Thus, although the subject of supervision appears within the nursing literature as a fairly consistent theme, there has been little or no attempt by the profession to give structure to either its underpinning theory or its practice. It is apparent that the term 'supervision' within the nursing profession has different meanings for different individuals and groups. In an attempt to explore the literature relating to the United Kingdom, the author has developed a structure for the review, based upon his reading of the literature and his own experience within the profession. The review covers five areas. The first area is that of examining the need for clinical supervision within the practice of nursing. The second area of the review identifies the various ways in which the concept of supervision is used in practice, particularly identifying the variety of terminology. The third area of the review is that of the profession's perception of good practice regarding supervision. The fourth area of the review seeks to identify various models of supervision as they are used within the nursing profession. Lastly, the preparation and training for the role of supervisor is reviewed.
Publication Types: Review; Review Literature

J Adv Nurs 1996 Nov;24(5):968-80
Models of differentiated practice and specialization in community nursing: a review of the literature.
Jansen PG, Kerkstra A, Abu-Saad HH, Van der Zee J.
Department of Nursing and Caring Research, Netherlands Institute of Primary Health Care (NIVEL), Utrecht, The Netherlands.
In most agencies for community nursing at least two types of nurse are employed. To ensure efficient use of personnel and high quality of nursing care, the principles of differentiated practice and specialization are used. It is suggested that these types of work redesign will have consequences for nurses and their work. We made a review of the literature to see how these principles are used and their effects on job satisfaction, burnout and quality of care. This review provides several views and descriptions of nursing activities, but it also shows that there is a paucity of quantitative data about the effects of differentiated practice and specialization in community nursing. To study these effects more systematically, a research model is presented. This model makes it possible to describe the changes in job characteristics caused by differentiated practice and

specialization. Secondly, it allows the effects on job satisfaction, burnout and quality of care to be studied.

J Adv Nurs 1996 Oct;24(4):682-7
The politics of collaboration as viewed through the lens of a collaborative nursing research project.
Beattie J, Cheek J, Gibson T.
Continuing Education Centre for Nurses, Queen Elizabeth Hospital, SA.
Collaborative research has much to offer nursing. However, the collaborative research process is fraught with issues arising from the 'politics of collaboration'. Such politics operate at the individual and institutional levels and can have debilitating effects on the research enterprise if they are not dealt with. This paper explores what is meant by collaboration and the politics of collaboration. Drawing on a critical perspective, it uses Brookfield's themes of impostorship, cultural suicide and roadrunning as the theoretical framework for the analysis. The paper uses an actual collaborative research project to ground the discussion provided.

J Adv Nurs 1996 Oct;24(4):800-9
Demand for post-qualifying professional education in the health care sector in England.
Calpin-Davies PJ.
SCHARR, Sheffield Centre for Health & Related Research, University of Sheffield, England.
The British National Health Service is proposing to establish local consortia for educational contracting, with the wider involvement and responsibility being devolved to service providers. This paper addresses the economic considerations of purchasing post-qualifying professional education in the English hospital sector, for hospital nurses, doctors and physiotherapists in England.

J Adv Nurs 1997 Nov;26(5):879-90
Emotional problems in primary care: what is the potential for increasing the role of nurses?
Mead N, Bower P, Gask L.
National Primary Care Research and Development Centre, University of Manchester, England.
It has been suggested that the role of primary care and community nurses should be expanded in relation to mental health in order to assist in the prevention and management of prevalent emotional disorders such as depression and anxiety. However, relatively little is known about the mental health work presently undertaken by these nurses. Furthermore, nurses' training needs, attitudes and organizational barriers to role expansion in this area have not been systematically explored. This article seeks to review the literature on nurses' potential and current mental health work, current and future training needs, the views of patients and nurses concerning an expanded nursing role, and organizational issues of relevance. Educational interventions which have been systematically evaluated are also reviewed. The results suggest that nurses are already involved in emotional health care with a variety of patient groups, although this is not always acknowledged as mental health work. While clear potential for an expanded role exists, there is little consensus as to what role would be most effective for each nursing group, and few educational interventions have been demonstrated to be of proven effectiveness.

J Adv Nurs 1997 Nov;26(5):946-52
Decision-making and paediatric pain: a review.
Abu-Saad HH, Hamers JP.
Department of Nursing Science, University Maastricht, The Netherlands.
h.huijer@vw.unimaas.rl
The aim of this paper is to present an overview of the literature on the factors influencing decision-making in the nursing care of children in pain. To that effect published and unpublished references were reviewed. The most frequently cited factors influencing the assessment and management of pain in children are summarized and discussed. Finally recommendations are made where further research is warranted.

J Adv Nurs 1998 Aug;28(2):391-7
Countertransference in the nurse-patient relationship: a review of the literature.
O'Kelly G.
St Michael's Hospital, Dunlaoghaire, Co. Dublin, Republic of Ireland.
Countertransference is a psychoanalytical concept which, when applied to nursing, refers to the unconscious response of the nurse to the patient. Psychoanalytical concepts such as the unconscious are infrequently mentioned in the nursing literature and have received little research attention. In this paper the literature about the nurse's countertransference is reviewed. In order that the psychodynamic aspects of this phenomenon are more fully appreciated, both the concepts of the unconscious and transference are first described. The nurse's countertransference has many expressions. The literature under review has highlighted the expression of countertransference through physical symptoms, through the nurse's level of involvement with the patient and through the nurse's positive and negative descriptions of patients. The value of recognizing countertransference is universally acknowledged. It is suggested that countertransference in the nurse-patient relationship should be explored further. The knowledge provided would help provide greater insights into the nurse-patient relationship, and ultimately will be reflected in the quality of care which the patient receives.

J Adv Nurs 1999 Mar;29(3):608-14
Assisting demented patients with feeding: problems in a ward environment. A review of the literature.
McGillivray T, Marland GR.
Acute/Rehabilitation Specialty, Crichton Royal Hospital, Dumfries, Scotland.
A critical review of the literature on assisting demented patients with feeding difficulties identifies that care at mealtimes is often task-centred, causing stress in both patients and staff and inadequate patient care. Nurses may even be inducing dependency in this vulnerable patient group. The staff to whom this care is most often delegated do not receive sufficient education or training to enable them to achieve a sufficient degree of empathy with the patient although there is evidence in the literature to suggest that this is a necessary requirement. It is also apparent that nurses use inadequate assessment criteria, perhaps due to the fact that there is an element of commonality in the feeding behaviour of demented patients which nurses feel they have seen many times and are able to deal with. The introduction of primary nursing, increased education of nursing assistants and improved assessment procedures to combat these problems are recommended. The process of change is briefly outlined and in conclusion some areas for future research are stated.

J Adv Nurs 2000 Dec;32(6):1325-32
Oral health care needs of dependent older people: responsibilities of nurses and care staff.
Fitzpatrick J.
Research in Health and Social Care Section, Florence Nightingale School of Nursing and Midwifery, King's College London, England.
joanne.fitzpatrick@kcl.ac.uk
The population of older people as well as the number of dependent older people is steadily increasing. Those unable to live independently at home are being cared for in a range of settings and varying degrees of dependency means that many are unable to attend fully to their needs, one aspect of which is oral care. The fact that the oral and dental health of the UK population is generally improving, makes more emphatic the responsibilities of nurses and care staff in this area. This review of the literature reveals that oral health of older people in continuing care settings is generally inadequate and that nurses' and care staff's knowledge and practice of oral care for older people is variable. Inadequate oral care is identified as multifactorial, with implications for educators, policy makers, practitioners and researchers. The need to address oral care for nurses pre- and post-registration as well as adequate preparation for support workers is highlighted. Development of a robust oral assessment

tool, as well as empirical investigation of the effectiveness of oral cleaning agents, equipment and techniques to inform standard setting is indicated, with monitoring of standards being imperative.

J Adv Nurs 2000 Mar;31(3):590-8
Mental health nurses and qualitative research methods: a mutual attraction?
Cutcliffe JR, Goward P.
Sheffield University and Royal College of Nursing Institute, Oxford, England.
Mental health nurses and qualitative research methods: a mutual attraction? In response to issues arising out of curriculum developments, the authors wished to examine more closely the potential reasons why psychiatric/mental health (P/MH) nurses appear to gravitate towards certain research methodologies. This paper therefore briefly examines the essential differences between qualitative and quantitative research paradigms, focusing on philosophical, epistemological and methodological issues. It then proceeds to examine some of the essential characteristics and attributes of P/MH nurses and suggests some differences in emphasis between these and other disciplines of nursing. The authors posit that psychiatric/mental health nurses are drawn to the qualitative paradigm as a result of the potential synchronicity and linkage that appears to exist between the practice of mental health nursing and qualitative research. This apparent synchronicity appears to centre around the three themes of: (a) the purposeful use of self; (b) the creation of an interpersonal relationship; and (c) the ability to accept and embrace ambiguity and uncertainty. Given this alleged synchronicity the authors argue that there are implications for nurse education and nursing research. Further it is possible that each nursing situation where the mental health nurse forms a relationship and attempts to gain an empathic sense of the individual's world is akin to an informal phenomenological study, the product of which would be a wealth of qualitative data. However, as this would be a subconscious, implicit process, the data would remain predominantly

unprocessed. The authors conclude that perhaps these data are the knowledge that expert practitioners draw upon when making intuition-based clinical judgements.

J Adv Nurs 2000 Nov;32(5):1298-306
Clinical supervision as an emancipatory process: avoiding inappropriate intent.
Heath H, Freshwater D.
School of Health Studies, Homerton College, Cambridge, England.
heath@health-homerton.ac.uk
As clinical supervision becomes more widely implemented in the United Kingdom with concerns and resistances being eroded as practitioners discover its benefits, it is important that potential limitations and perhaps failures are avoided. This paper utilizes Johns' (1996) intent-emphasis axis to explore how a technical interest, misunderstanding of expert practice, and confusion of self awareness with counselling, can detract from the supervisory process. Several of the criticisms of reflective practice will be examined to demonstrate where concerns are valid and where they may be based on misunderstandings and the need to control clinical supervision. Greater awareness of inappropriate emphasis and intent should enable even relatively inexperienced supervisors to help their supervisees move towards independence, emancipation and evolving expertise.

J Adv Nurs 2000 Oct;32(4):975-80
Backstage in the theatre.
Tanner J, Timmons S.
School of Health Care Studies, University of Leeds, England. j.a.tanner@leeds.ac.uk
Observations undertaken in the operating theatre suggested that the social environment, and certain forms of staff behaviour could be explained using the space analysis developed by Erving Goffman (1969) in The Presentation of Self in Everyday Life. In the study reported in this paper the theatre department was found to be a strongly 'backstage' area. However, it was also found that there were limits to this analysis, and these are explained within this article. Some

practical suggestions as to how this analysis might be helpful in the management of health care institutions and the education of health care professionals are made.

J Adv Nurs 2001 Sep;35(5):674-82
Action research from the inside: issues and challenges in doing action research in your own hospital.
Coghlan D, Casey M.
Lecturer in Business Studies, School of Business Studies, University of Dublin, Trinity College, Dublin, Ireland.
david.coghlan@tcd.ie
BACKGROUND AND RATIONALE: Nurses are increasingly engaging in action research projects to improve aspects of nursing practice, education and management and contribute to the development of the profession. Action research involves opportunistic planned interventions in real time situations and a study of those interventions as they occur,. which in turn informs further interventions. Insider action research has its own dynamics which distinguish it from an external action researcher approach. The nurse-researchers are normally already immersed in the organization and have a pre-understanding from being an actor in the processes being studied. There is a paucity of literature on the challenges that face nurse action researchers on doing action research in their own hospital. AIM: The aim of this article is to address this paucity by exploring the nature of the challenges which face nurse action researchers. Challenges facing such nurse-researchers are that they frequently need to combine their action research role with their regular organizational roles and this role duality can create the potential for role ambiguity and conflict. They need to manage the political dynamics which involve balancing the hospital's formal justification of what it wants in the project with their own tactical personal justification for the project. MAIN ISSUES: Nurse-researchers' pre-understanding, organizational role and ability to manage hospital politics play an important role in the political process of framing and selecting their action research project. In order that the action research project contribute to the organization's learning, nurse action researchers engages in interlevel processes engaging individuals, teams, the interdepartmental group and the organization in processes of learning and change. CONCLUSIONS: Consideration of these challenges enables nurse-action researchers to grasp the opportunities such research projects afford for personal learning, organizational learning and contribution to knowledge.

J Am Diet Assoc 1997 Oct;97(10 Suppl 2):S131-8
Charting by exception: a solution to the challenge of the 1996 JCAHO's nutrition care standards.
Charles EJ.
Marriott Management Services, Atlantic City Medical Center, NJ 08401, USA.
With charting by exception, only significant findings or exceptions to the norms are documented in script by the nursing staff. Upon admission, patients are screened for nutrition risk or need for nutrition education by nursing staff using an interdisciplinary patient database. Patients with predetermined criteria indicating nutritional risk or with nutrition education needs are referred to nutrition services. Using specified criteria, the clinical nutrition staff assign referred patients to a level of care. Nutrition care or education is provided and documented within 48 hours. Documentation varies with the level of nutrition care.

J Burn Care Rehabil 2001 May-Jun;22(3):250-4; discussion 249
Management of an inpatient-outpatient clinic an eight-year review.
Yurko LC, Coffee TL, Fusilero J, Yowler CJ, Brandt CP, Fratianne RB.
Department of Nursing, MetroHealth Medical Center, Case Western Reserve, University School of Medicine, Cleveland, Ohio 44109-1998, USA.
Healthcare organizations have historically separated outpatient from inpatient facilities. In order to streamline the

continuity of high quality care, an outpatient burn clinic was established on our inpatient burn center in 1991. Management of the outpatient clinic required alternate staffing patterns and supply allocation plus training in managed care and third party payors. Budget decisions and health care trends affected the number of full time equivalents (FTEs). Between 1990 and 1998, a 33% RN FTE reduction occurred with an overall 22% decrease in total inpatient care providers. Clinic positions were allocated as patient volume and workload data could justify additional staff. Enhanced flexibility in assignment and use of personnel with varying skill levels led to efficient integration of inpatient and outpatient care with an overall reduction in RN FTEs. The purpose of this study is to review the changes in nursing management strategies required by this consolidation.

J Burn Care Rehabil 2001 May-Jun;22(3):250-4; discussion 249
Management of an inpatient-outpatient clinic an eight-year review.
Yurko LC, Coffee TL, Fusilero J, Yowler CJ, Brandt CP, Fratianne RB.
Department of Nursing, MetroHealth Medical Center, Case Western Reserve, University School of Medicine, Cleveland, Ohio 44109-1998, USA.
Healthcare organizations have historically separated outpatient from inpatient facilities. In order to streamline the continuity of high quality care, an outpatient burn clinic was established on our inpatient burn center in 1991. Management of the outpatient clinic required alternate staffing patterns and supply allocation plus training in managed care and third party payors. Budget decisions and health care trends affected the number of full time equivalents (FTEs). Between 1990 and 1998, a 33% RN FTE reduction occurred with an overall 22% decrease in total inpatient care providers. Clinic positions were allocated as patient volume and workload data could justify additional staff. Enhanced flexibility in assignment and use of personnel with varying skill levels led to efficient

integration of inpatient and outpatient care with an overall reduction in RN FTEs. The purpose of this study is to review the changes in nursing management strategies required by this consolidation.

J Child Fam Nurs 1999 Mar-Apr;2(2):82-9; discussion 89-91; quiz 92
Culturally competent nursing research: are we there yet?
Villarruel AM.
University of Pennsylvania, School of Nursing, Philadelphia, USA.

J Child Health Care 1998 Spring;2(1):31-5
Dispelling modern day myths about children's pain.
Twycross A.
University of Central England, Edgbaston, Birmingham.
Children are still enduring unnecessary pain. Nurses and other health care professionals continue to believe the misconceptions about paediatric pain which contribute to this. These misconceptions have all been shown to have no scientific basis.

J Child Health Care 1998 Summer;2(2):80-5
Influences on nurses' perceptions of children's pain.
Twycross A.
University of Nottingham, School of Nursing, Postgraduate Division, Queen's Medical Centre.
Individuals have their own perceptions of pain. Nurses' do not always perceive their patients' pain. There are a number of factors which influence nurses' perceptions of their patients' pain. Further research is needed in this area.

J Child Health Care 1998 Winter;2(4):178-81
Clinical education in pediatrics.
James E.
Kent and Canterbury Hospital.
The clinical environment is an important factor in the student nurse's learning experience. The literature identifies a number of key areas which form the clinical learning environment. The reality of the ward environment and the literature demonstrate gaps between theory and

practice. Ongoing evaluation of the ward environment could increase the learning opportunities available to Students

J Clin Nurs 1996 Mar;5(2):121-5
Nursing the physically disabled in a general hospital ward.
Conway K.
Progress in medical treatment over the last three decades has meant that many more people survive either traumatic birth situations or diseases/injuries which would have previously resulted in death, and are leading normal lives with some form of physical disability. Until quite recently, little attention has been given to their longer-term health needs. The following article looks at the attitudes of nurses towards physically disabled patients, the experiences and attitudes of these patients, the interaction between nurse and patient, practical outcomes and future directions. Literature on this subject is not extensive. More empirical research is required focusing on the impact of admission of such people on general hospital ward functioning, the experiences/insights of nursing staff caring for them and the reaction and comments of physically disabled patients.

J Clin Nurs 1997 May;6(3):173-8
Clinical supervision.
Goorapah D.
Faculty of Health and Social Care, University of the West of England, Education Centre, Royal United Hospital, Combe Park, Bath, UK.
The introduction of clinical supervision to a wider sphere of nursing is being considered from a professional and organizational point of view. Positive views are being expressed about adopting this concept, although there are indications to suggest that there are also strong reservations. This paper examines the potential for its success amidst the scepticism that exists. One important question raised is whether clinical supervision will replace or run alongside other support systems.

J Clin Nurs 1998 May;7(3):218-26
Nursing development units: their structure and orientation.
Redfern S, Stevens W.
Nursing Research Unit, King's College London.
This paper provides background material about the Department of Health funded Nursing Development Units (NDUs), specifically their biographical and contextual characteristics, their aims and values, and their organization of work and resources acquired. The data were drawn from questionnaires to clinical leaders and from documentation. The findings are summarized under five questions which address the NDUs' values and aims, their organization of work, multiprofessional working, activeness in acquiring resources and support and the effect of the host organization. Taken as a whole, the aims match the vision of the ideal NDU specified by the pioneers of the NDU movement, and most clinical leaders subscribed to primary nursing as their preferred mode of organizing nursing work. Multiprofessional working was a common feature and there was considerable evidence of equality in team membership status. A small number of NDUs had been awarded grants for research and most were successful in generating income from conferences. Nearly all had links with an academic institution. NDUs that had the support of their Trust's management were able to market their services successfully. Our findings indicate that many NDUs have made good progress but their clinical leaders are the first to admit that there is much more to be done.

J Clin Nurs 1999 Jan;8(1):22-30
Nursing assessment and diagnosis of respiratory distress in infants by children's nurses.
Armitage G.
School of Health Studies, University of Bradford, UK.
Many children's nurses have significant contact with children who have breathing difficulties and should be using systematic criteria to assess their nursing needs.

Children's nurses do not appear to follow systematic criteria but are strongly influenced by the medical model and this may be detrimental to holistic assessment and the development of nursing diagnoses based on nursing needs. As nursing, along with other disciplines, develops evidence-based practice, children's nurses should develop evidence for best practice mindful of children's views, parental needs and the education of future practitioners.

J Clin Nurs 1999 Jul;8(4):338-44
The effectiveness of a group approach to clinical supervision in reducing stress: a review of the literature.
Williamson GR, Dodds S.
Institute of Health Studies, University of Plymouth, UK.
There is little research evidence to suggest that clinical supervision reduces stress. However, this probably does not mean that clinical supervision is not valuable, just that the evidence is not yet there, because consensus exists that group clinical supervision may be beneficial in reducing stress in nurses. The work by Butterworth et al. is the only directly relevant study investigating the stress-reducing potential that a group approach to clinical supervision has, and this work establishes ground rules for future evaluation.
Publication Types: Review; Review Literature

J Clin Nurs 1999 Sep;8(5):496-504
Factors contributing to medication errors: a literature review.
O'Shea E.
Beaumont Hospital, Dublin 9, Ireland.
Drug administration is an integral part of the nurse's role. Responsibility for correct administration of medication rests with the nurse, yet medication errors are a persistent problem associated with nursing practice. This review examines what constitutes a medication error and documents contributory factors in medication errors. These factors have been derived from reported medication errors and opinions of nurses as to factors which predispose to errors. A number of definitions exist as to what constitutes a medication error. The

definition used should facilitate interpretation and comparison of a wide range of research reports. Medication errors are a multidisciplinary problem and a multidisciplinary approach is required in order to reduce the incidence of errors.
Publication Types: Review; Review Literature

J Contin Educ Nurs 1996 Jul-Aug;27(4):168-75; quiz 192
Research utilization and the continuing/staff development educator.
Mottola CA.
Current health care imperatives and the continuous explosion of information and technology present new challenges for continuing/staff development educators as the nursing profession reinvents itself during the current crisis in health care. This turbulent health care environment necessitates utilization of current research findings to maintain the continued efficient and effective functioning of nursing staff. Familiarity with recent research utilization projects and models and barriers perceived to impede research utilization can assist the continuing/staff development educator to bridge the gap between knowledge generation and knowledge utilization.

J Contin Educ Nurs 1996 Sep-Oct;27(5):209-14
Reflective learning: work groups as learning groups.
Carkhuff MH.
Clinical Information System, York Health System, Pennsylvania, USA.
Staff development educators are challenged to develop additional learning strategies to meet the demands of the professional nurse in the changing healthcare environment today. Methodology for workplace learning is being developed to meet the critical thinking skills necessary for the professional nurse of the future. This article identifies the use of reflective learning in the workplace and reports outcomes from the implementation of the reflection-on-action technique. The implications for staff development educators are reviewed for the concept of

work groups as learning groups.

J Contin Educ Nurs 1996 Sep-Oct;27(5):215-9
Critical Path education: necessary
components and effective strategies.
Aronson B, Maljanian R.
Division of Nursing Education and
Research, Hartford Hospital, Connecticut
06102-5037, USA.
Proper use of Critical Paths based on a
solid educational foundation aids
caregivers in meeting the ultimate
challenge of today's healthcare
environment: to provide a higher quality of
care at a lower cost. The components for a
comprehensive educational program for
Critical Paths include general principles,
Path contents, Path development,
guidelines for documentation, variance
data collection and evaluation. A strategy
to provide large numbers of staff with
background information is through the use
of self-learning packets; the case study
approach is an appropriate strategy for Path
specific education. Evaluation data indicate
that both strategies are effective in
assisting staff to develop and implement
Critical Paths.

J Contin Educ Nurs 1997 Jan-Feb;28(1):26-31
Nurses and Public Law 102-119: a family-
centered continuing education program.
Winstead-Fry P, Bishop KK.
School of Nursing, University of Vermont,
Burlington 05405, USA.
The passage of Part H of the Education of
the Handicapped Act, Public Law 99-457,
and the reauthorization of the law in 1991,
as Public Law 102-119, mandates a family-
centered approach to the provision of
services to infants and young children with
handicaps. Nurses are named as providers
in this federal legislation. The authors
conducted a survey to assess the learning
needs of nurses who may wish to serve as
providers under the law. The survey results
were used to develop a family-centered
continuing education curriculum that pairs
parents and nurse faculty as partners in
delivering the curriculum.
Publication Types: Review; Review
Literature

J Contin Educ Nurs 1997 Jul-Aug;28(4):150-6
Thinking about thinking.
Ulsenheimer JH, Bailey DW, McCullough
EM, Thornton SE, Warden EW.
Carolina Medicorp, Inc., Winston-Salem,
North Carolina, USA.
BACKGROUND: The nursing leadership
at a 900-bed tertiary-care facility in the
southeast believed an opportunity existed
to improve the critical thinking abilities of
the professional nursing staff.
METHOD: A team, consisting of a
diversified group of nurse educators and
managers, had the opportunity to gain
understanding of the critical thinking
process of the nursing staff as well as to
develop a plan designed to improve critical
thinking skills.
RESULTS: Outputs of the team included
development of a critical thinking model
and process as well as an action plan that
specifically outlined how it would
implement the model within the
organization using a preceptor-based
educational process.
CONCLUSION: Nursing leadership within
this facility believes that nurturing critical
thinking in the staff will have a positive
impact on care delivery outcomes. Creating
shared visions through the assumptions
that the staff and organization hold is
important to improving care provided.
Assisting staff with using a critical
thinking process in order to construct, tear
down, and then reconstruct clinical
incidents as encouraged by this model is
one key to problem-solving.

J Contin Educ Nurs 1997 Jul-Aug;28(4):181-7
Collaborative research among clinical
nurse specialists and staff nurses.
Govoni AL, Pierce LL.
Cleveland State University Department of
Nursing, Ohio, USA.
BACKGROUND: Conducting research in
clinical settings can be problematic for
many nurses in practice due to lack of
experience and support.
METHOD: Research collaboration
between clinical nurse specialists and staff
nurses in clinical settings can promote
development of their research process
skills.

RESULTS: Strategies identified can be applied by clinical nurse specialists involved in continuing education and staff development in clinical practice through further research development. CONCLUSION: Collaboration among clinical nurse specialists and staff nurses provides a unique and strong link that transcends degrees and roles to make substantial contributions to professional nursing practice.

J Contin Educ Nurs 1997 Mar-Apr;28(2):64-8
Patient stories: a way to enhance continuing education.
Stamler LL, Thomas B.
School of Nursing, University of Windsor, Ontario, Canada.
Using breast health and illness, this article reviews relevant research literature and compares it for congruency with patient stories. Inconsistencies and issues found are related to desired outcomes and decision-making. Patients may view cancer treatment as an unbroken continuum from pre-diagnosis to completion of treatment. While moving through the continuum, they interact with nursing professionals in several roles and locations. Strategic suggestions acknowledge the need to incorporate health professionals, patients and families in the continuing education activity. Nurses working in continuing education have the opportunity to improve care along the treatment continuum and reduce the distance between research and practice. Implications for nursing practice and continuing education are identified. Suggestions for enhancing continuing education related to this continuum are made.
Publication Types: Review; Review Literature

J Contin Educ Nurs 1997 Sep-Oct;28(5):211-6
Identification, intervention and education: essential curriculum components for chemical dependency in nurses.
Pullen LM, Green LA.
University of Tennessee, Knoxville 37922, USA.
BACKGROUND: A documented need exists for continuing education in the area of chemical dependency as it relates not only to patient care, but also to nurses who are susceptible to addiction. This is significant due to the fact that nurses are at risk for chemical dependency and many nurse peers are unable to recognize the signs of chemical dependency and therefore unable to actively intervene. CONCLUSION: According to the literature, which includes current research, nurses lack knowledge regarding specific risk factors, symptoms of chemical dependency in peers, and steps for intervention. In addition, the literature revealed that nursing curricula allot little time to chemical dependency issues. The results of a small-scale learning needs assessment support this literature finding. Continuing education courses can effectively educate nurses to be able to identify their own susceptibility and those of chemically dependent peers, intervene appropriately, and begin the healing process for the impaired nurse. This article outlines a curriculum and additional resources to address the learning needs of nurses related to chemical dependency.

J Contin Educ Nurs 1997 Sep-Oct;28(5):231-4
Gaming: a teaching strategy to enhance adult learning.
Henry JM.
Wellesley Central Hospital, Toronto, Ontario, Canada.
BACKGROUND: As a nurse educator, I encountered many complaints from staff nurses about mandatory inservice education programs, stating that they are repetitious, time-consuming, often too basic, and at times, downright boring. One exception was an Infection Control Week education session that was done in the form of a game. This session set attendance records and had very positive feedback from staff nurses. As a result of this feedback, the use of gaming as a teaching strategy in nursing education was explored. METHOD: A review of the literature on gaming as a teaching strategy was conducted with special attention to its history, current use, and successes in nursing education. RESULTS: Introduced as a formal

teaching strategy more than 75 years ago, gaming offers many advantages over more traditional teaching methods. Games connect theory more closely to real life situation and add innovation, diversity, and the opportunity for immediate feedback. Although gaining in popularity, gaming is not extensively used in nursing education as it is not considered a serious educational tool. However, recent literature suggests much success with its use. CONCLUSION: Gaming as a teaching strategy has proven to be an effective way of conveying information in a stimulating, appealing manner. Games facilitate both beginning and experienced nurses' learning by providing an opportunity for experience without the danger or fear of jeopardizing patient safety.

J Contin Educ Nurs 1998 May-Jun;29(3):105-11
Using role theory concepts to understand transitions from hospital-based nursing practice to home care nursing.
Murray TA.
University of Missouri-St. Louis, College of Nursing 63121, USA.
BACKGROUND: The phenomena experienced by professional nurses who make practice-based career changes are seldom addressed in the literature. Nurses changing from a hospital-based practice to a home health care setting report feelings of anxiety, incompetency, and lack of the necessary skills to care for clients in the home.
METHOD: An integrative review of the literature on role theory can provide the conceptual understanding of the transitional experience of nurses whose roles change when they move from hospital-based practice to a home health care setting.
RESULTS: A model of the role transition process is helpful in identifying the transition experienced by nurses new to the home health care setting. Experiences during the initial transition period are critical in shaping the nurse's understanding of the role.
CONCLUSION: Educators can play a key part in assisting novice home health care

nurses with role enactment by developing comprehensive orientation and education programs aimed at minimizing role strain.

J Contin Educ Nurs 1998 Sep-Oct;29(5):211-6
A review of preceptorship in undergraduate nursing education: implications for staff development.
Letizia M, Jennrich J.
Loyola University Chicago, Maywood, IL 60153, USA.
Nurse educators regularly develop clinical learning experiences for undergraduate students using the expertise of experienced RNs as preceptors. Preceptors help students develop a knowledge base and clinical skills. This article reports a literature review and summarizes the benefits of preceptorship, outlines preceptor responsibilities and qualities, and discusses the process of preceptor selection and role preparation. Suggestions for collaborative efforts regarding the preceptor experience among staff nurses, nurse educators, and staff development educators are highlighted.

J Contin Educ Nurs 1998 Sep-Oct;29(5):221-7
The use of gaming strategies in a transcultural setting.
Gary R, Marrone S, Boyles C.
Center for Distance Learning, King Faisal Specialist Hospital and Research Center, Riyadh, Saudi Arabia.
Saudi Arabia's vast economic resources have enabled the development of state-of-the-art hospitals. Nurses recruited from around the world staff these hospitals creating one of the most multicultural practice settings in the world. Ethnic, educational, and experiential diversity; language and communication barriers; and alternative ways of knowing and learning challenge nurse educators to be more creative and explore opportunities for greater participation and learning among various cultural groups. Gaming, as a teaching-learning strategy for multicultural participants, affords the necessary flexibility and nonthreatening atmosphere which facilitates positive interactions among different, and often competing, communication patterns and learning

styles. This article explores how and why gaming is as an effective educational strategy in a transcultural setting.

J Contin Educ Nurs 1999 May-Jun;30(3):105-7; quiz 142-3
Preparing staff to deliver age-appropriate nursing care to elderly patients.
Travis SS, Duer B.
Oklahoma Center on Aging, University of Oklahoma Health Sciences Center, Oklahoma City 73190, USA.
Meeting the Joint Commission on Accreditation of Healthcare Organizations accreditation standard for age-appropriate care cannot be accomplished by a once-a-year inservice educational program. Educational offerings that address the specialty of gerontological nursing require deliberate decision-making regarding the generic and advanced competencies necessary for care of elderly patients. Finding the resources to effectively teach the essential (generic and advanced) content is challenging. This article suggests that a staff development department may use existing resources and personnel from other organizations to prepare nursing staff to deliver age-appropriate care to elderly patients.

J Contin Educ Nurs 1999 May-Jun;30(3):140-1
Genetics 101 essential for all nurses.
Foote P.

J Contin Educ Nurs 1999 May-Jun;30(3):140-1
Genetics 101 essential for all nurses.
Foote P.

J Cult Divers 1998 Winter;5(4):138-46; quiz 147-8
Workforce diversity and cultural competence in healthcare.
Shaw-Taylor Y, Benesch B.
Westat, Inc., Rockville, Maryland, USA.
This paper presents a discussion of workforce diversity in healthcare and its attendant requisite of cultural competency. The first section of the paper argues that self-assessments and diversity training are integral to workforce diversity management. This paper maintains that diversity training should be a part of overall strategic goals, and that the development of management goals should be based on self-assessments. The second section of the review offers a framework of cultural competency in healthcare delivery based on the relationship between patient and provider, and the community and health system. For this relationship to be successful, this review argues that health systems should foster providers that can also be cultural brokers. The cultural broker role is seen as core to achieving cultural competency.

J Emerg Nurs 1996 Aug;22(4):317-22
Update on nursing employment.
Zimmermann PG.

J Emerg Nurs 1996 Aug;22(4):317-22
Update on nursing employment.
Zimmermann PG.

J Emerg Nurs 2000 Aug;26(4):312-7
The use of unlicensed assistive personnel: an update and skeptical look at a role that may present more problems than solutions.
Zimmermann PG.
Department of Nursing, Harry S Truman College, Chicago, Ill., USA.
pzimmermann@ccc.edu
Patients implicitly rely on nurses to be their advocate. They trust nurses for health care information (92%). Approximately three fourths of Americans rated nurses' honesty and ethics as either "high" or "very high", placing them above any other profession. It is time to reconsider the full implication of Florence Nightingale's admonition to do the sick no harm in terms of staffing.
Publication Types: Review; Review Literature

J Gerontol Nurs 1997 Feb;23(2):31-40
Research-based practice: reducing restraints in an acute care setting--phase I.
Cruz V, Abdul-Hamid M, Heater B.
University of Iowa College of Nursing, Iowa City, USA.
The purpose of this research utilization project was to select and implement a research-based Restraint Education Program for reducing the use of restraints

in an acute care setting by changing the perception of the restraint coordinators about restraints in the direction of decreased importance. The Iowa Model, Research Based Practice to Promote Quality Care (Titler et al., 1994) was selected to guide the change process. A multidisciplinary team reviewed the restraint policy and procedure, new restraint products and alternative restraint methods. After a review of the literature on restraint education programs, the committee concluded that education was the key component in decreasing the use of physical restraints. The research-based Restraint Education Program developed by Drs. Strumpf and Evans was selected as the educational program. Education sessions were developed and a pilot study was conducted with the restraint coordinators. The Perceptions of Restraint Use Questionnaire (PRUQ) (Strumpf & Evans, 1988) was administered before and after the education sessions. The results of the t-test showed a decrease in the post-test mean scores on 7 of the 17 items indicating a less important perception by the staff about the use of restraints. Four items had an increase in mean scores on the post-test indicating the restraint coordinators increased their perception of the importance of physical restraints with these items. The restraint education program was presented to the nursing staff throughout the institution. Risk management and quality assurance will monitor patients restrained and evaluate the nursing staff with the PRUQ in 3 months.
Publication Types: Review; Review Literature

J Hosp Infect 2000 Oct;46(2):96-105
Educating the infection control team - past, present and future. A British prespective.
Jenner EA, Wilson JA.
Faculty of Health and Human Sciences, University of Hertfordshire, Hatfield, Hertfordshire, UK.
E.A.Jenner@herts.ac.uk
This review sets out to explore how education and training provisions for members of the Infection Control Team (ICT) have developed alongside their roles and in response to changes in the British National Health Service. It focuses on the Consultant in Communicable Disease Control, the Infection Control Doctor and the Infection Control Nurse in the United Kingdom, but also briefly considers approaches adopted by other countries. Future developments should include maximizing information technology for delivering teaching materials, shared learning and improvements to pre-registration curricula for both doctors and nurses. Copyright 2000 The Hospital Infection Society.

J Intraven Nurs 1997 Mar-Apr;20(2):89-93
Nurses transition from hospital to home: bridging the gap.
Coulter K.
Coulter Consulting in Clearwater, Florida, USA.
Practice transition between health care settings is often fraught with frustration, stress, and even traumatic learning experiences for nurses. As the need for qualified infusion therapists in home care increases, more acute care nurses are making the transition from hospital to home. This article is designed to profile the differences between the care settings and offer suggestions to smooth the change from hospital to home care.

J Neurosci Nurs 1998 Aug;30(4):220-4
Pharmacological management of pain after intracranial surgery.
Leith B.
Montreal Neurological Hospital, Intensive Care Unit, Quebec, Canada.
Some healthcare professionals continue to believe that patients experience minimal pain and discomfort after intracranial surgery. However, clinical experience indicates that many patients experience significant pain after craniotomy. Despite research which supports the use of morphine as a method of pain control after intracranial surgery, some healthcare professionals continue to administer only codeine, which may be ineffective. Inadequate pain control can be associated with a variety of negative physiological

and psychological consequences. Neuroscience nurses are challenged to re-evaluate their current beliefs and practices related to pain and pain control after intracranial surgery.

J Nurs Adm 1996 Mar;26(3):38-46
Integration of emerging designs for the practice and management of nursing.
Blouin AS, Tonges MC.
Ernst & Young, LLP, Chicago, Illinois, USA.
Work redesign and shared governance represent two of the most popular administrative innovations in contemporary nursing. Whereas work redesign creates changes in the content of nurses' jobs, shared governance addresses the organizational context within which nurses are employed. Although the content and context of nurses' work are closely interrelated, many organizations have attended to one of these issues, but failed to give consideration to the other. Building on this background, the state of the art in nursing redesign and restructuring is summarized, and emerging directions in job and organizational design are identified.

J Nurs Adm 2000 Jul-Aug;30(7-8):347-50
Job satisfaction and nurses in rural Australia.
Hegney D, McCarthy A.
University of Southern Queensland, Australia.

J Nurs Adm 2001 Apr;31(4):179-86
The nursing shortage revisioning the future.
Purnell MJ, Horner D, Gonzalez J, Westman N.
School of Nursing, University of Miami, USA. mpurnell@miami.edu
A severe shortage of nurses is being experienced nationally and globally. In South Florida, one of the most severely impacted regions in the world, a group of healthcare organizations, educational institutions, and nursing organizations formed the Nursing Shortage Consortium to combat the nursing shortage. Strategic efforts to recruit and retain nurses are

underway, with a focus on nurturing interest among young people and increasing opportunities to stimulate their interest, to increase the supply of appropriately prepared professional nurses.

J Nurs Adm 2001 Apr;31(4):179-86
The nursing shortage revisioning the future.
Purnell MJ, Horner D, Gonzalez J, Westman N.
School of Nursing, University of Miami, USA. mpurnell@miami.edu
A severe shortage of nurses is being experienced nationally and globally. In South Florida, one of the most severely impacted regions in the world, a group of healthcare organizations, educational institutions, and nursing organizations formed the Nursing Shortage Consortium to combat the nursing shortage. Strategic efforts to recruit and retain nurses are underway, with a focus on nurturing interest among young people and increasing opportunities to stimulate their interest, to increase the supply of appropriately prepared professional nurses.

J Nurs Adm 2001 Jul-Aug;31(7-8):346-52
Instruments for evaluating nurse competence.
Meretoja R, Leino-Kilpi H.
Helsinki University Central Hospital, Finland. riitta.meretoja@hus.fi
Publication Types: Review; Review, Academic

J Nurs Care Qual 2001 Jul;15(4):48-59
Quality measures essential to the transformation of the Veterans Health Administration: implications for nurses as co-creators of change.
Valentine NM.
Nursing Strategic Healthcare Group, Department of Veterans Affairs, Washington, DC, USA.
Health care systems are changing at an unprecedented rate, but few are making the changes in a system affecting nearly 200,000 staff in over 1,100 different sites of service delivery originating from 171 medical centers nationwide, as is the Veterans Health Administration. The

issues of change, quality of care, morale and opportunities involved in being a nurse today in a system undergoing this magnitude of change is presented within the framework of the quality of care initiatives that have been launched by VA. The new organization design of VA, emphasizing local decision-making, a description of the multiple quality programs recently introduced and integrative strategies that have been used by the Nursing Strategic Healthcare Group, the VA corporate level policy and nursing programs information center for the country, to support the change process are discussed.

J Nurs Manag 1996 Sep;4(5):297-300
The nursing profession and its relationship with hospital managers.
Rickard NA.
This paper describes the relationship between the professional nursing and managerial imperatives in health care and explains some of the ways the managerial culture affects the working environment of professional nurses. It goes on to highlight some of the professional developments of the last 17 years and describes how these could augment the difference in imperatives. Finally it suggests ways in which the nursing profession might develop to maintain its unique contribution to health care, whilst embracing the managerial domain. This is necessary to ensure that professional nursing is nurtured and not overwhelmed by workloads and empirical assessments of nursing outputs.

J Nurs Manag 1997 Jan;5(1):43-50
Do nurses really care? Some unwelcome findings from recent research and inquiry.
Fletcher J.
Department of Nursing and Midwifery Studies, Queens Medical Centre, Nottingham, UK.
This paper examines the position of nursing as a caring profession, in terms of an ethical code that stresses collegial relationships, a sense of obligation to a clientele that is realized in terms of expert service, and a clearly defined body of research-derived knowledge as the basis

for practice. It also investigates the substance of the claim that nursing has tended to arrogate to itself another operational distinction-its exclusive capacity to blend physical and emotional support into care. A review of recent research and investigation, undertaken in a number of countries, suggests that nursing as practiced, rather than as theorized, fails to fulfil its wider professional aspirations, and to fulfil its caring rhetoric. A related paper will consider how the absorption of nursing into higher education might begin to play a part in developing and consolidating the professionalization of nursing.

J Nurs Manag 1997 May;5(3):167-73
Job diagnostic surveys of paediatric nursing: an evaluative tool.
Eaton N, Thomas P.
Department of Nursing, Midwifery and Health Care, University of Wales, Swansea, UK.
Two distinct trends can be identified in the context within which nursing care is planned and delivered. One is the continuous pressure to find ways of increasing efficiency and cost-effectiveness. The second is the widespread expectation that public services in general, and health services in particular, should be monitored and evaluated. In these circumstances, nurses and their managers need a range of evaluative tools so that changes in the organization of nursing care can be evaluated. Hackman and Oldham's 'Job Diagnostic Survey' (JDS) approach was tested in a Paediatric Unit in which aspects of primary nursing were being introduced. The paper outlines the JDS approach in the Unit in question and offers an assessment of the value of the JDS as an evaluative tool.

J Nurs Manag 1998 May;6(3):165-72
Measuring the unmeasurable: a caring science perspective on patient classification.
Fagerstrom L, Engberg IB.
Faculty of Social and Caring Sciences, Abo Akademi University, Vasa, Finland.
AIMS: To give a short historical survey of

patient classification and its motives, to analyse patient classification and especially the instrument, The Oulu Patient Classification more closely from a caring science perspective.
BACKGROUND: A survey of topical literature and research on patient classification show that economic and administrative justifications predominate and the caring science connection is weak, almost non-existent.
ORIGINS OF INFORMATION: Topical literature and research on patient classification and the instrument, The Oulu Patient Classification.
DATA ANALYSIS: Topical literature and research were evaluated from a caring science perspective in accordance with Eriksson's theory of caring and the basic concept of man as an entity of body, soul and spirit.
KEY ISSUES: Patient classification is used in staff planning and is also justified from the viewpoint of content, that is, as a method of guaranteeing good quality in the care of patients and as an expression of the prevalent caring ideology. The concept of man is reduced in current literature and research on patient classification. The Oulu Patient Classification is based on a humanistic view of man, but man's spiritual and existential needs do not emerge clearly from the manual of the instrument.
CONCLUSIONS: It is essential for patient classification to start from a caring perspective. Correctly dimensioned staffing based on patient classification is a prerequisite for good care. This should be combined with a caring culture that considers the whole complexity of man in order to make good care possible.

J Nurs Manag 1999 Jan;7(1):13-7
Our healthier hospital? The challenge for nursing.
Robinson SE, Hill Y.
Centre for Health Education and Research, Canterbury Christ Church University College, UK.
AIM: This paper aims to explore the problems which are currently preventing hospital nurses from fulfilling their health promotion role, and makes recommendations for nursing managers.
BACKGROUND: Hospital nurses have a key role to play in meeting recent Government proposals, which aim to enhance health promotion and public health in the NHS.
KEY ISSUES: Lack of knowledge and skills, unhealthy hospital environments, poor collaboration, insufficient time and poor nursing management are impediments to hospital nurses promoting health.
CONCLUSIONS: Hospital nurse managers need to capitalize on government enthusiasm by supporting health promotion education for nursing staff improving the hospital environment and facilitating better interdisciplinary working.

J Nurs Manag 1999 Jul;7(4):193-200
Shared governance: time to consider the cons as well as the pros.
Gavin M, Ash D, Wakefield S, Wroe C.
Department of Social Work, University of Salford, Manchester, UK.
AIMS: This paper aims to provide a critical appraisal of an approach to the management and organization of nursing work known as shared governance (SG).
BACKGROUND: This approach has its origins in the USA, where, during the past 20 years it has become increasingly influential. The advocates of SG claim that it can, inter alia, improve recruitment and retention rates, boost morale, and help raise clinical skills. Little wonder that SG in now beginning to make significant inroads into the NHS.
ORIGIN OF INFORMATION: However, a trawl through the extensive US literature, using printed and online (e.g. BIDS, CINHAL, MEDLINE, etc.) bibliographical sources, suggests that the claimed benefits of SG should be treated with caution.
KEY ISSUES: Much of the existing published research appears to be both methodologically flawed and lacking in any critical edge. While many researchers and commentators appear only too willing to highlight what they see as the promise of SG, they shy away from exploring any potential pitfalls. One consequence of this is that many of the putative benefits SG is

said to confer, may in fact be more apparent than real.

CONCLUSIONS: Nurses and nurse managers need to be apprised of and consider seriously, the possible cons as well as the potential pros of SG, if any promise it may have is to be realized.

Publication Types: Review; Review Literature

J Nurs Manag 1999 Nov;7(6):339-47

Promoting quality of care for older people: developing positive attitudes to orking with older people.

Wade S.

Oxford Brookes University School of Health Care, John Radcliffe Hospital, Headington, UK.

AIMS: Managers and administrators have a key strategic role and responsibility or the way the care of older people is delivered within health and social care services, since the decisions made and directions taken at this level have a direct influence on services delivered. This article provides an outline of the context in which the services provided for older people have emerged, especially within health care, and offers strategies for the way forward. BACKGROUND: The standard of care received by older people is high on the agenda in contemporary health care. Frequent reports have questioned this quality over the years, yet concerns still remain. A key factor influencing quality of care received by older people, can be attributed to the persistence and perpetuation of ageist attitudes held by society and those working within health and social care settings at all levels. METHODS: Drawing upon a range of literature, an overview of those factors that seem to be attributable to the development of contemporary attitudes and perceptions about older people and their care are reviewed, focusing particularly upon health and social care workers, especially nurses. FINDINGS: The role of education in particular is explored as this has a key role in influencing attitudes towards caring for older people and will impact directly on the way in which all care and services develop.

CONCLUSION: A number of areas are outlined for future development and research that aim to address and serve the needs of older people, and which could be supported at a managerial and administrative level to promote positive attitudes.

J Nurs Manag 1999 Sep;7(5):265-70

Identifying, evaluating and implementing cost-effective skill mix.

Richardson G.

Centre for Health Economics, University of York, UK.

BACKGROUND: The British National Health Service (NHS) employs a large number of individuals, at great monetary cost, to provide direct care to patients. Changes in the combinations of staff, including nurses, nurse practitioners and midwives, delivering this care have been shown to be effective in many settings. FINDINGS: The (opportunity) cost implications of such changes in the skill mix are rarely evaluated adequately. The impact of releasing professionals' time has not been estimated and therefore determining whether changes are cost-effective is difficult; these difficulties have often been increased by poor study design. CONCLUSIONS: Economic evaluation has been under-utilized in studies of skill mix. If economic evaluation demonstrates that skill mix changes reduce cost and improve or maintain patient outcomes, this is strong evidence that these changes should be implemented. Incentives may be required to attract the necessary personnel. This in itself may influence the cost of changing the skill mix and therefore the situation should be monitored as both costs and effectiveness can alter over time.

J Nurs Manag 2000 Mar;8(2):115-20

Enrolled nurse conversion: a review of the literature.

Webb B.

Postgraduate Education Centre, Princess Marina Hospital, Northampton, UK.

AIM: The aim of this literature review was to examine the policies and professional literature from the last 50 years about the introduction, the role and subsequent plight of the enrolled nurse (also known as second level nurses), and the need to convert to the first level of the UKCC nursing register.

BACKGROUND: Nurse shortages within the NHS have been cyclical since its inception in 1948. The policy decision to cease the training of enrolled nurses within the frame of modernizing the education and training of the nursing workforce had two distinct implications for enrolled nurses. Firstly, they could choose to stay as enrolled nurses or convert to first level nursing. Nevertheless, enrolled nurses have cited the lack of funded conversion course places, and managerial support for non-conversion.

METHODS: A critical review of the national policies and professional literature concerned with the evaluation of enrolled nurses' contribution to the NHS.

FINDINGS: It was argued that national policy needs to be supported on the ground, whereby enrolled nurses are proactively supported to come forward for conversion and/or meaningful roles are created and sustained where enrolled nurses continue to make a valuable contribution to the NHS agenda. Finally, the paper challenges all NHS organizations to consider the profile and value of enrolled nurses and become proactive in their recruitment and retention of this nursing group.

Publication Types: Review; Review Literature

J Nurs Staff Dev 1996 May-Jun;12(3):127-32
Working with lesbian, gay, and bisexual people. Reducing negative stereotypes via inservice education.
Eliason MJ.
Basic components of an inservice program that concerns working with lesbian, gay, and bisexual people are presented. Staff nurses will encounter such people in every nursing specialty and will have lesbian, gay, and bisexual coworkers whether they know it or not. Inservice programs that deal with any sexuality issue must include cognitive and affective interventions, because negative or uncomfortable attitudes may have been ingrained since

childhood.

J Nurs Staff Dev 1997 Jul-Aug;13(4):193-7
Action research applied to a preceptorship program.
Balcain A, Lendrum BL, Bowler P, Doucette J, Maskell M.
Women's Health & Wellness Consultants, Burlington, Ontario, Canada.
In this article the authors describe the development of a framework designed to discuss expectations between preceptors, orientees, nursing unit managers and clinical nurse educators. Action research theory provided the framework for this process. Preceptors found the process of articulating expectations helpful, relevant, and meaningful to their practice.

J Nurs Staff Dev 1997 Mar-Apr;13(2):67-72
Environmental Protection through waste management, Implications for staff development.
Cox M, Rhett C, Gudmundsen A.
Rome Group, Incorporated, Arlington, Texas, USA.
Increasing public concern is focusing on healthcare providers as a primary source of medical waste. As nurses practice in expanded roles in a variety of settings, attention must be paid to teaching them how to be ecologically responsible by assessing the environmental impact of the services they provide and providing ways to reduce the volume of waste.

J Nurs Staff Dev 1997 May-Jun;13(3):119-24
Pain, role play, and videotape. Pain management staff development in a community hospital.
Daroszewski EB, Meehan DA.
Granada Hills Community Hospital, California, USA.
Videotaped role play was an effective staff development strategy used as an initial exercise in a five-part class to update the pain management skills of experienced nurses. It engaged the participants in learning and stimulated discussion and provided concrete feedback of current clinical practices for comparison with the Agency for Health Care Policy and Research pain management guidelines

(Acute Pain Management Guideline Panel, 1992).
Publication Types: Review; Review Literature

J Nurs Staff Dev 1997 May-Jun;13(3):126-30
Implementing effective staff education about advance directives.
DesRosiers M, Navin P.
University of Massachusetts Medical Center (UMMC), Worcester, USA.
The Patient Self-Determination Act of 1990 guarantees the right to refuse medical or surgical treatment and the right to draft advance directives. This review of the current literature provides those in nursing staff development and inservice education with an overview of advance directives and their implications for nursing education and practice. Possible core subjects for inclusion in planned, purposeful, advance directive education programs are examined, including cultural sensitivity, facilitator skills, interviewing techniques, legal information, patient autonomy, and reasoning and decision making. This review provides a platform for future research.

J Nurs Staff Dev 1997 May-Jun;13(3):149-54
Level of literacy in the nurses aide population. Baseline data for nursing staff development.
Benjamin BA.
College of Nursing, Rutgers, State University of New Jersey, Newark, USA.
A study of literacy levels of the nurses aide population working in selected acute-care hospitals showed that a literacy deficit existed, described the type and degree of the deficit, and determined its prevalence according to selected demographic factors. Implications for staff development educators in roles of orientation, inservice, and continuing education are discussed for this population in regard to current changes in healthcare delivery patterns.
Publication Types: Review; Review Literature

J Nurs Staff Dev 1997 May-Jun;13(3):155-60
Word games as a cost-effective and innovative inservice method.

Stringer EC.

J Nurs Staff Dev 1997 May-Jun;13(3):163-9
Evaluation of an orientation system for newly employed registered nurses.
Straub CW, Mishic B, Mion LC.
Department of Education and Research, Cleveland Clinic Foundation, Ohio, USA.
In this article, the authors discussed the successful evaluation of an orientation system for newly employed registered nurses in a large teaching hospital using the IOP model. This methodology can be successfully applied to any educational program that is consolidated into an organization's goals. Although not well examined, orientation has been reported to be costly (Bethel, 1992; del Bueno, Weeks, Brown-Stewart, 1987). The system presently used at this hospital uses at least 1 week of a nurse educator's time, 3-10 weeks for a newly employed registered nurse, and 3-10 weeks for a preceptor RN. Such an investment of personnel resources mandates examination of the processes and outcomes of the program to ensure newly employed RNs become competent practitioners as efficiently as possible. The use of the IOP model particularly was useful in examining a complex orientation system in a multicentered hospital. Use of this systematic program evaluation separated the overall orientation process into workable components. Tools, such as the algorithm, allowed for easy visualization and comprehension of the process steps. This was indispensable because of the number and scope of people involved in the orientation program. The evaluation process was impartial and focused on the program steps, not on the individuals. Because of this impartiality, people were able to gather and work cohesively to improve the overall program. Use of the IOP model assisted the nurse educators in determining that PBDS was not achieving the goal of identifying individual learning needs. Rather, PBDS was a useful tool in establishing baseline competency of newly employed RNs. The system clearly identified those individuals who had above average knowledge bases and those individuals who had more

learning needs. For those with more learning needs, PBDS provides a starting point for planning a structured orientation. Thus, a Phase II PBDS assessment could be used as a more unit-specific assessment to validate whether the RN has achieved the orientation objectives. Although the IOP model is not a strict research methodology, it is appropriate for examination of a program as fluid and ongoing as this. Finally, ongoing run charts or statistical trends will assist the nurse educators in monitoring the quality and effectiveness of the orientation program.

J Nurs Staff Dev 1997 May-Jun;13(3):163-9
Evaluation of an orientation system for newly employed registered nurses.
Straub CW, Mishic B, Mion LC.
Department of Education and Research, Cleveland Clinic Foundation, Ohio, USA.
In this article, the authors discussed the successful evaluation of an orientation system for newly employed registered nurses in a large teaching hospital using the IOP model. This methodology can be successfully applied to any educational program that is consolidated into an organization's goals. Although not well examined, orientation has been reported to be costly (Bethel, 1992; del Bueno, Weeks, Brown-Stewart, 1987). The system presently used at this hospital uses at least 1 week of a nurse educator's time, 3-10 weeks for a newly employed registered nurse, and 3-10 weeks for a preceptor RN. Such an investment of personnel resources mandates examination of the processes and outcomes of the program to ensure newly employed RNs become competent practitioners as efficiently as possible. The use of the IOP model particularly was useful in examining a complex orientation system in a multicentered hospital. Use of this systematic program evaluation separated the overall orientation process into workable components. Tools, such as the algorithm, allowed for easy visualization and comprehension of the process steps. This was indispensable because of the number and scope of people involved in the orientation program. The evaluation process was impartial and focused on the program steps, not on the individuals. Because of this impartiality, people were able to gather and work cohesively to improve the overall program. Use of the IOP model assisted the nurse educators in determining that PBDS was not achieving the goal of identifying individual learning needs. Rather, PBDS was a useful tool in establishing baseline competency of newly employed RNs. The system clearly identified those individuals who had above average knowledge bases and those individuals who had more learning needs. For those with more learning needs, PBDS provides a starting point for planning a structured orientation. Thus, a Phase II PBDS assessment could be used as a more unit-specific assessment to validate whether the RN has achieved the orientation objectives. Although the IOP model is not a strict research methodology, it is appropriate for examination of a program as fluid and ongoing as this. Finally, ongoing run charts or statistical trends will assist the nurse educators in monitoring the quality and effectiveness of the orientation program.

J Nurses Staff Dev 1998 Jul-Aug;14(4):169-75
The nurse educator role in the clinical setting.
Mateo M, Fahje CJ.
Department of Nursing, Mayo Clinic, Rochester, Minnesota, USA.
mmateo@mayo.edu
Although educators in clinical settings assume different roles, the major responsibilities are the clinical and professional development of staff. Some of the challenges facing educators relate to maintaining expertise, maintaining visibility, and managing work load. In this article, the authors describe the responsibilities of the educator and the challenges and strategies for success in the clinical educator role.

J Nurses Staff Dev 1998 Jul-Aug;14(4):183-7
Improving critical thinking in nursing practice.
Fowler LP.
Department of Health Promotion, Medical University of South Carolina, Florence,

USA.
Nurse educators and practicing nurses agree that the complexity of health care demands critical thinking skills. In this article, the author describes critical thinking and its development both as knowledge based and practice bound. Included are strategies nurses can use to further develop critical thinking skills. Case scenarios are presented for educators to consider in promoting nurses' reflection and clinical reasoning skills in their practice settings.

J Nurses Staff Dev 1998 Nov-Dec;14(6):267-72
Critical thinking. Strategies for clinical practice.
Bittner NP, Tobin E.
Regis College, Weston, Massachusetts, USA.
Critical thinking is an elusive concept. As a profession, nursing has yet to accept a universal definition of critical thinking. Despite the lack of consensus, nurse leaders in academia and practice settings overwhelmingly agree that critical thinking is essential. It is clear, considering the healthcare environment, nurses need to use critical thinking as a process for decision making in the clinical arena. This article clarifies critical thinking in practice by illuminating the imperative role it plays. Suggestions for fostering critical thinking, including specific strategies, provide a framework for practice.

J Nurses Staff Dev 1998 Nov-Dec;14(6):283-5
Documentation in the land of perfect charts. How to turn your frogs into princes.
Webster MR.
Total Care, Inc., Charlotte, North Carolina, USA.
In this article, the author describes an innovative approach to teaching adult learners. A theatrical atmosphere was used with medieval characters, music, and head gear. This class about documentation was designed to spur creativity, team work, and ultimate individual accountability.

J Nurses Staff Dev 1998 Sep-Oct;14(5):240-3
Teaching managed care to hospital staff.
Haggard A.
Huntington Hospital, Pasadena, California, USA.
Meeting the challenge of providing managed care information to hospital staff necessitates a creative approach to content and teaching techniques. Examples are provided for selecting information to be taught and methods for presenting it in a way that encourages participation and follow through in the workplace. Evaluation involves evaluating the quantity and quality of ideas generated by the learners, as well as visiting different departments to ensure implementation of those ideas.

J Nurses Staff Dev 2000 Jan-Feb;16(1):23-30
Facilitating critical thinking.
Hansten RI, Washburn MJ.
Hansten & Washburn, Bainbridge Island, Washington, USA.
Supporting staff to think effectively is essential to improve clinical systems, decrease errors and sentinel events, and engage staff involvement to refine patient care systems in readiness for new care-delivery models that truly reflect the valued role of the RN. The authors explore practical methods, based on current research and national consulting experience, to facilitate the development of mature critical thinking skills. Assessment tools, a sample agenda for formal presentations, and teaching strategies using behavioral examples that make the important and necessary link of theory to reality are discussed in the form of a critical thinking test as well as a conceptual model for application in problem solving.

J Obstet Gynecol Neonatal Nurs 1997 May-Jun;26(3):320-6
Comment in: J Obstet Gynecol Neonatal Nurs. 1998 Mar-Apr;27(2):125
Patient-focused models of care.
Pence M.
Women's & Children's Services, John Muir Medical Center, Walnut Creek, CA 94598, USA.
The structure and the process for delivering

patient care will experience major changes during the next decade. Most hospitals have tried different alternatives, including restructuring, re-engineering, redesign, and the return to patient-focused care. Staffing strategies may successfully move nurses from total patient care to delegated, shared accountability. During their short stays, new parents and their neonates receive streamlined, intensely focused care from cross-trained workers in a patient-focused care environment. Each interaction becomes a meaningful and educational one, with the focal point being the mother and the family.

J Obstet Gynecol Neonatal Nurs 2001 Mar-Apr;30(2):209-15
Culturally competent care of women and newborns: knowledge, attitude, and skills.
Callister LC.
Brigham Young University College of Nursing, Provo, UT 84602-5544, USA. lynn_callister@byu.edu
In a variety of health care settings throughout the United States and Canada, nurses are caring for women and newborns from culturally diverse backgrounds. In the technologically complex and bureaucratic world of health care delivery, cultural considerations in provision of care often are overlooked and neglected. The purpose of this article is to define ways in which culturally competent nursing care can be implemented. Nursing education and clinical practice guidelines are clear on the importance of gaining cultural competence. Providing culturally competent care includes understanding the dimensions of culture; moving beyond the biophysical to a more holistic approach; and seeking to increase knowledge, change attitudes, and hone clinical skills. Building on the strengths of women rather than utilizing a deficit model of health care is an essential part of providing culturally competent care. The achievement of both measurable and "soft" outcomes related to the delivery of culturally competent care can make a critical difference in the heath and well-being of women and newborns.

J Obstet Gynecol Neonatal Nurs 2001 May-Jun;30(3):269-74
The importance of the sexual health history in the primary care setting.
Peck SA.
Nurses often are apprehensive when inquiring about women's sexual health issues. A comprehensive sexual health assessment, however, is an important part of the health history and interview. Ensuring confidentiality and maintaining professionalism will create the trusting, comfortable environment necessary for a thorough evaluation of a client's sexual health risks. Nurses who are familiar with diverse sexual issues can help women deal with the changes that may occur during the life span.

J Perianesth Nurs 1997 Apr;12(2):109-12
The problem with accountability.
Muller-Smith P.
Department of Education at Saint Francis Hospital, Tulsa, OK., USA.
Accountability is an issue that creates stress and frustration for managers at all levels within an organization. With the current trends to "push decision-making down" and "empower people" to run more efficient units or departments, many managers are finding most of their efforts are not yielding the intended results. Employees are not embracing new responsibilities and accountability. They seem to find it another burden added to what they report as already too much work. What can be done to manage this dilemma? Interestingly enough, the solution may have to start by taking a journey into self-awareness.

J Perianesth Nurs 1997 Aug;12(4):289-92
Learning to learn: step one for survival in the new paradigm.
Muller-Smith P.
Department of Education, Saint Francis Hospital, Tulsa, OK, USA.
New challenges require new approaches and many of the suggested solutions are in conflict with how we were taught in our formative years. Team work in high school and college was mostly found in sports-related activities. Collaboration in a

classroom was not encouraged and could be viewed as cheating. We did not learn to share knowledge in a group nor to group problem solving, yet we are told that those are the very skills we need to have to survive in today's workplace. The first step to success is to look at how we were taught to learn and make the shift to learning in a different manner.

J Perianesth Nurs 1998 Aug;13(4):250-2
The game may be the same but the rules have changed!
Muller-Smith P.
Saint Francis Hospital, Tulsa, OK, USA.
The job of a manager continues to be one of achieving outcomes through other people. However, in the current work environment, managers are finding that while their scope of responsibility is expanding, the traditional power base used to excourage high performance is shrinking. There are limited rewards a manager can use to gain commitment from their staff. Even if some of those rewards are available, many of the new employees do not see them as motivators. Employees come to the workplace with a different set of expectations. There seems to be a mismatch between the traditional management approach to getting the best from the worker and what the worker wants from their manager. In as much as the workplace and the worker are changing so too must manager's approach to "getting the job done."

J Perianesth Nurs 1998 Jun;13(3):191-5
Power shift: creating an empowered workforce.
Muller-Smith P.
Department of Education, Saint Francis Hospital, Tulsa, OK 74136, USA.
To do more with less requires being able to empower others so that they are accountable and responsible. In many situations, staff resist empowerment and often make comments to the effect that it is the manager's job to get certain things done--not theirs! In moving toward empowerment, the most difficult first step must be a personal step to gain insight into the type of power the manager uses to

achieve outcomes. If in the process of self-examination they find that their personal style of power does not support empowerment, then they must first make a power shift to a style that creates an environment where staff empowerment can be accomplished.

J Perianesth Nurs 1998 Oct;13(5):317-9
Being the boss is not what it used to be!
Muller-Smith P.
Department of Education, Saint Francis Hospital, Tulsa, OK, USA.
Mentoring has a long and varied history. It was a method for helping people grow to competence in a supportive environment. As being a boss continues to have less and less real power associated with the role, the idea of approaching employees as partners in getting the work accomplished makes the concept of mentoring applicable to today's workplace and today's workforce.

J Perinat Neonatal Nurs 2000 Mar;13(4):13-30
The process of triage in perinatal settings: clinical and legal issues.
Mahlmeister L, Van Mullem C.
Birth Center, San Francisco General Hospital, California, USA.
The process of triage in perinatal settings often has been considered the sole function of the labor and delivery nurse. In fact, all nurses have a legal and professional duty to engage in the systematic identification of patient-client problems, prioritization of needs, and prompt deployment of personnel and equipment to meet those needs. In-person and telephone triage occur in all obstetric ambulatory and acute care settings. The organized steps in triage should be identical regardless of the location or size of the perinatal service. The redesign of women's and neonatal services, the reduction of professional nursing staff, and predictions of a growing nursing shortage require perinatal nurses to develop highly refined triage skills.

J Pract Nurs 1998 Jun;48(2):16-9
Every nurse is a leader.
Fisher L, Davidhizar R.
Some nurses have the goal to lead others and to be in charge of patient groups and

groups of staff. They want to make changes at the upper levels of the organization and see their actions affect large numbers of people. Many others, however, really desire to be a bed-side nurse giving excellent patient care. They want to enjoy the close relationship that can make an individual feel better about him or her self as a person and the satisfaction that they have made a difference in one person's life. However, whether the nurse leads through a management position or practices leadership techniques in bedside nursing, all nurses are leaders and need to demonstrate expertise in the use of leadership techniques.

J Pract Nurs 2000 Summer;50(2):16-8; quiz 19, 22
The art of getting what you want for optimal patient care.
Davidhizar R.
Getting your way is a mix of logical and emotional issues. It is important to establish rapport and meet a person emotionally before trying to sell an idea. It is essential to think an idea through clearly ahead of time and to present it clearly and logically. The possibility of resistance should be anticipated so that the presentation addresses potential areas of resistance. It is important to actively listen, to agree when possible, and to not appear too eager. Persuasion is both an art and science. When used skillfully, persuasive techniques are powerful tools of communication and productivity.

J Prof Nurs 1998 Jul-Aug;14(4):242-53
Differentiated levels of nursing work force demand.
Kovner CT, Schore J.
Division of Nursing, School of Education, New York University, New York 10012, USA.
In addition to reviewing the literature about the extent to which basic nursing education is related to actual nursing practice, this article investigates the extent to which the relationship between nursing practice, education, and experience varies across specific health care settings. The literature presented no consistent or systematic association between type and amount of previous nursing experience and current nursing practice. However, the literature generally provided evidence of a consistent and systematic association between baccalaureate preparation and level of registered nurse (RN) practice. The review of practice and organizational differences across the hospital, nursing home, and ambulatory care sectors suggests that baccalaureate-prepared RNs in hospitals may have a more strongly differentiated role relative to those in nursing homes and ambulatory settings. If baccalaureate-prepared nurses continue to be perceived as capable of more complex and independent practice, and if employers believe that they can increase revenues by increasing the quality of nursing care or can save money by shifting to RNs some responsibilities now held by more costly personnel (such as physicians), then demand for baccalaureate-prepared nurses may increase.

J Psychiatr Ment Health Nurs 1997 Apr;4(2):125-9
Mentoring state hospital nurses to write.
Davidhizar R, Cosgray R.
Bethel College, Mishawaka, Indiana, USA.
There is a shortage of clinical nurses, particularly in the area of psychiatric nursing, who feel competent and comfortable writing for publication. This is unfortunate since clinical nurses have valuable experiences to share, to promote and advance the nursing profession. This manuscript describes the work of one Director of Nursing at a state hospital who mentored the nursing staff to write for publication. Over a period of five years some 28 articles have been published by nurses at this hospital. This success in publication has led to an increase in self-esteem among nurses, an increased willingness to share their writing experiences with others, and increased numbers of workshop presentations on clinical subjects. This article describes how the mentoring process can be used to promote authorship, and specifically, how

it was used at this one hospital.

J Psychiatr Ment Health Nurs 1998
    Oct;5(5):361-5
    Intensive care psychiatric nursing--
    psychoanalytic perspectives.
    Winship G.
    Psychotherapy Department, West
    Berkshire NHS Trust, Reading, UK.
    Based on unobtrusive observations, a
    parallel is drawn between general and
    psychiatric intensive care nursing. The
    correlation between bedside skills and the
    incidence of physical contact between
    nurse and patient in each setting is
    considered. The phenomenon of physical
    attacks by patients on carers and the
    process of restraint in the psychiatric
    intensive care unit (ICU) is then examined.
    It is suggested that attack by and
    subsequent restraint of a disturbed patient
    may be considered in terms of an
    unconscious re-enactment of an early skin-
    on-skin object relation. It is argued that the
    physical holding of a psychotic patient is
    functional in re-establishing their bodily
    ego. Some thoughts are offered on how the
    intensive care of psychotic patients might
    be carried forward in the future.

J Psychiatr Ment Health Nurs 1999
    Apr;6(2):101-6
    Psychological needs of patients with HIV
    disease: reviewing the literature using
    Nichols' (1985) Adjustment Reaction
    Model as a framework.
    Murphy M, Melby V.
    Heartlands Hospital, Birmingham, UK.
    Since the first manifestations of HIV
    infection presented in the United Kingdom
    in the early 1980s, there has been a
    dramatic increase in the incidence of HIV
    infection and a proliferation of diseases
    associated with HIV infection. HIV
    infection is now associated with physical,
    psychological, mental and neurological
    conditions. Many of these conditions are
    serious and pose a major threat to physical
    and mental health, with rapid deterioration
    of health status necessitating multiple
    hospital admissions to acute hospitals. The
    majority of people hospitalized with HIV
    diseases are currently being cared for on
    general wards. While physical needs are
    often well met, psychological needs are to
    a certain extent neglected. The literature
    cites numerous cases of neglect,
    discrimination and threats to
    confidentiality by health professionals,
    including nurses. Such psychological
    needs, emanating out of hospitalization,
    compound existing psychological needs.
    Nichols' (1985) Adjustment Reaction
    Model describes a number of stages
    patients may go through during the course
    of their illness, and to some extent the
    patient's psychological needs can be traced
    throughout the trajectory of the disease.
    The purpose of this paper is to review the
    literature and present a theoretical
    argument, using Nichols' model as a
    framework, on psychological needs of
    patients with HIV diseases, and attempt to
    outline to what extent psychological needs
    of patients with HIV are met in
    institutional care. The authors recommend
    further research to determine nurses'
    perception of the importance of meeting
    psychological needs of patients with HIV
    disease.
    Publication Types: Review; Review
    Literature

J Psychiatr Ment Health Nurs 1999
    Feb;6(1):15-20
    Triumvirate nursing for personality
    disordered patients: crossing the
    boundaries safely.
    Melia P, Moran T, Mason T.
    Personality Disorder Unit, Ashworth
    Hospital, Liverpool, UK.
    As the issue of the treatment and effective
    management of personality disordered
    patients comes under close scrutiny in the
    wake of the Fallon Inquiry, we offer a brief
    overview of the nature of the challenges
    involved in nursing this difficult group of
    patients. Traditional methods of setting
    limits and defining boundaries are no
    longer convincing amidst the allegations of
    multidisciplinary staff being culpable, at
    one level or another, for their contribution
    in this tragic inquiry. In this paper we offer
    a strategic mechanism of constructing
    nursing care for this difficult group of
    patients and provide a framework for

crossing boundaries safely through a multidisciplinary framework. We term this triumvirate nursing. Nursing management of those patients considered to have personality disorders is traditionally very difficult. This difficulty, in part, stems from the inability of nurses to strategically develop therapeutic relationships in a safe manner. Crossing boundaries is a necessary part of therapeutic exploration and relationship building; triumvirate nursing offers a safe mechanism for undertaking this. Creative thinking is a necessary part of the future development of the nursing management of these disorders.

J Psychiatr Ment Health Nurs 2000 Jan;7(1):7-14

Stress and burnout in community mental health nursing: a review of the literature.
Edwards D, Burnard P, Coyle D, Fothergill A, Hannigan B.
School of Nursing Studies, University of Wales College of Medicine, Heath Park, Cardiff, UK.
There is a growing body of evidence that suggests that many community mental health nurses (CMHNs) experience considerable stress and burnout. This review aimed to bring together the research evidence in this area for CMHNs working within the UK. Seventeen papers were identified in the literature, seven of which looked at stress and burnout for all members of community mental health teams (CMHTs) and the remaining 10 papers focused on CMHNs. The evidence indicates that those health professionals working as part of community teams are experiencing increasing levels of stress and burnout as a result of increasing workloads, increasing administration and lack of resources. For CMHNs specific stressors were identified. These included increases in workload and administration, time management, inappropriate referrals, safety issues, role conflict, role ambiguity, lack of supervision, not having enough time for personal study and NHS reforms, general working conditions and lack of funding and resources. Areas for future research are described and the current study of Welsh CMHNs is announced.

This review has been completed against a background of further significant changes in the health service. In the mental health field, specific new initiatives will have a significant impact on the practice of community mental health nursing. A new National Framework for Mental Health, along with a review of the Mental Health Act (1983), will undoubtedly help to shape the future practice of mental health nursing.
Publication Types: Review; Review Literature

J R Soc Med 2001;94 Suppl 39:9-12
Improving quality measures in the emergency services.
Armitage M, Flanagan D.
Bournemouth Diabetes and Endocrine Centre, Royal Bournemouth Hospital, Castle Lane East, Bournemouth BH7 7DN, UK. mary.armitage.@rbch-tr.swest.nhs.uk
A large and continuing increase in medical emergency admissions has coincided with a reduction in hospital beds, putting the acute medical services under great pressure. Increasing specialization among physicians creates a conflict between the need to cover acute unselected medical emergencies and the pressure to offer specialist care. The shortage of trained nursing staff and changes in the training of junior doctors and the fall in their working hours contribute to the changing role of the consultant physician. The organization of the acute medical service is of paramount importance and requires multi-disciplinary teamwork on an admissions unit with full support services. Excellent bed management is essential. There must be guidelines for all the common medical emergencies and all units must undertake specific audits of the acute medical service. Continuing professional development (CPD) and continuing medical education (CME) should reflect the workload of the physician; that is, it must include time specifically focused on acute medicine and general (internal) medicine, as well as the specialty interest.

J Rural Health 1991;7(4 Suppl):402-12
Future trends in nursing practice and

technology.
Fuszard B.
School of Nursing, Medical College of
Georgia, Augusta 30912.
Rural hospitals will be affected by changes
in nursing anticipated in the future.
Welcome changes will be the maturity and
life experiences new graduates will bring
to the work setting, knowledge of
computers, and a broadening database.
New graduates will also know various
methods of care delivery, including case
management, and will be able to select the
delivery system that best meets the needs
of the patients and institution. They will be
more autonomous and possess leadership
and management skills. With their
knowledge of community as well as
institutional nursing, they will be able to
draw upon the skills of both groups to
bring the two areas of nursing into
continuity of care for patients. A difficulty
ahead for rural hospitals is recruitment of
new graduates, the majority of whom will
have established families and lives
elsewhere. And the practice of developing
their own employees for higher levels of
nursing will be compounded by the
doubling of time necessary to complete
nursing programs in the future.

J UOEH 1996 Sep 1;18(3):239-45
[Occupational dangers to health of nursing
staffs in hemodialysis units]
[Article in Japanese]
Washio M, Utoguchi K, Mizoue T,
Yoshimura T.
Department of Clinical Epidemiology,
University of Occupational and
Environmental Health, Kitakyushu, Japan.
Since hemodialysis patients are at high risk
for blood-borne viral infection such as
hepatitis B and C virus infection, nursing
staffs of the hemodialysis units have a
significant occupational exposure to blood-
borne virus infection. Furthermore, they
are in danger of contacting occupational
low back-pain because they have to take
care of patients in a half-rising position. In
addition, they may also suffer from
burned-out syndrome because they have to
look after all the chronic renal failure
patients as well as run machines during the
hemodialysis procedure. In this paper, we
describe occupational danger to health of
nursing staffs working in hemodialysis
units.

J Wound Care 1997 May;6(5):244-7
Comment in: J Wound Care. 1997
May;6(5):207
Knowledge base and use in the
management of pressure sores.
Maylor ME.
Pembrokeshire NHS Trust, Haverfordwest.

J Wound Care 1998 Apr;7(4):211-2
Wound assessment methods.
Banks V.
Cardiff Community Healthcare Trust, UK.

J Wound Care 1998 Jan;7(1):21-3
The classification of pressure sores.
Banks V.
Dip Community Health Studies, Cardiff
Community Healthcare Trust, UK.

J Wound Care 1998 Jul;7(7):369-70
Management issues in pressure area care.
Banks V.
Cardiff Community Healthcare NHS Trust,
UK.

J Wound Care 1998 May;7(5):265-6
Pressure sores: topical treatment and the
healing process.
Banks V.
Cardiff Community Healthcare Trust, UK.

J Wound Care 1999 Jun;8(6):291-4
Comment in: J Wound Care. 1999
Jun;8(6):267
Wound debridement, Part 2: Sharp
techniques.
Vowden KR, Vowden P.
Bradford Royal Infirmary, UK.

J Wound Ostomy Continence Nurs 1997
Jan;24(1):19-25
Effects of a pressure-reduction mattress
and staff education on the incidence of
nosocomial pressure ulcers.
Boettger JE.
St. Joseph's Regional Health Center, Hot
Springs, Arkansas 71913, USA.
PURPOSE: The purpose of this study was

to determine whether replacing standard hospital mattresses with pressure-reduction mattresses and educating the patient care team on Agency for Health Care Policy and Research prevention guidelines would decrease the incidence of nosocomial pressure ulcers.

DESIGN: Retrospective chart review before and after implementation of replacement of standard hospital mattresses with pressure-reduction mattresses and before and after patient care team education was completed.

SETTING AND SUBJECTS: A 6-month clinical study with 141 subjects was conducted on a skilled-nursing unit.

METHODS: The 3-month preintervention sample group of 141 subjects received routine nursing care on a standard hospital mattress. After the introduction of pressure-reduction mattresses and an education program, a 3-month postintervention sample group of 141 subjects was studied.

MAIN OUTCOME MEASURES: Incidence of nosocomial pressure ulcers during a 3-month period.

RESULTS: Among the preintervention group, 21 of 141 subjects (15%) acquired nosocomial pressure ulcers, versus 16 of 141 subjects (11%) in the postintervention group. This improvement was not statistically significant (chi 2 = 0.78, df = 1, p = 0.38). The incidence of ulcers staged II or higher dropped from 11 patients in the preintervention group to six in the postintervention group. A 45% reduction that was not statistically significant (chi 2 = 1.56, df = 1, p = 0.21).

CONCLUSION: Replacement of standard hospital mattresses and education of staff according to recommendations from the Agency for Health Care Policy and Research guideline for pressure ulcer prediction and prevention did not significantly change the incidence of pressure ulcers during a 3-month period in our skilled-nursing unit.

Publication Types: Review; Review Literature

Lippincotts Prim Care Pract 1999 Mar-Apr;3(2):216-28; quiz 228-30

Acute symptom assessment: determining the seriousness of the presentation.
Fletcher K, Forch W.
Geriatric Division, University of Virginia, Charlottesville, USA.

Nursing home residents are typically frail elders of advanced age who have comorbidities and are taking multiple medications. These residents are particularly vulnerable to acute illness and often demonstrate this illness in an atypical fashion. Nursing home staff need to be skilled in the recognition of acute illness and exacerbations of chronic illness in the resident so that expeditious assessment and management of disease or illness is ensured. The clinician with advanced skill in symptom and sign assessment and management strategies is better prepared to make an accurate diagnosis and to teach the nursing staff the critically needed observation and assessment skills.

Med Care 1997 Oct;35(10 Suppl):OS13-25
Hospital restructuring in the United States, Canada, and Western Europe: an outcomes research agenda.
Sochalski J, Aiken LH, Fagin CM.
Center for Health Services and Policy Research, School of Nursing, University of Pennsylvania, Philadelphia 19104-6096, USA.

OBJECTIVES: This article describes the extent and nature of hospital restructuring across the United States, Canada, and Western Europe, countries with differently organized and financed health-care systems, and assesses the feasibility of international research on the outcomes of hospital restructuring.

METHODS: The conceptual background, context, and focus for the Bellagio conference on Hospital Restructuring in North America and Western Europe held in November 1996 is provided, illustrating key issues on hospital and workforce trends using the US data with international comparisons.

RESULTS: Hospital systems internationally are undertaking very similar restructuring interventions, particularly ones aimed at reducing labor expenses through work redesign. Nursing has been a

prime target for work redesign, resulting in changes in numbers and skill mix of nursing staff as well as fundamental reorganizing of clinical care at the inpatient unit level. Yet little is known about the outcomes of such organizational interventions and there are few efforts in place to critically evaluate these actions. CONCLUSIONS: Restructuring of the hospital workforce and redesign of work in inpatient settings is widespread and markedly similar across North American and Europe, and warrants systematic study. Cross-national studies of the impact of restructuring inpatient care on patient outcomes would yield valuable lessons about the cost-quality tradeoffs in hospital redesign and re-engineering, as well as inform national planning about the numbers and types of nurses needed in the coming decades.
Publication Types: Review Review, Tutorial

Med Care 1997 Oct;35(10 Suppl):OS1-4
Evaluating the consequences of hospital restructuring.
Aiken LH, Fagin CM.
Center for Health Services and Policy Research, School of Nursing, University of Pennsylvania, Philadelphia 19104-6096, USA.

Med Care 1997 Oct;35(10 Suppl):OS7-12
Hospital restructuring in North America and Europe.
White KL.

Medsurg Nurs 1997 Apr;6(2):90-4
Medication calculation skills of the medical-surgical nurse.
Ashby DA.
Columbia Suburban Hospital, Louisville, KY, USA.
Medication administration is one of the most time-consuming aspects of nursing practice. Expertise in medication calculation and administration is essential to the treatment of all patients; however, many nurses experience difficulty when calculating medications. In this study, 56.4% of nurses could not calculate medications correctly in 90% of the

problems, suggesting the need for regular self-testing of medication calculation skills. Continuing education programs implemented for identified medication calculation errors influences nursing practice and patient care outcomes.
Publication Types: Review; Review Literature

Medsurg Nurs 1997 Dec;6(6):350-3, 356-8
Inserting and maintaining peripherally inserted central catheters.
Driscoll M, Buckenmyer C, Spirk M, Molchany C.
Lehigh Valley Hospital, Allentown, PA, USA.
Peripherally inserted central catheters are a type of vascular access device that has many advantages for patients with longer-term and special infusion needs. Increasingly common in home and hospital settings, nurses should know how to insert, maintain, and educate patients and families about these devices. One hospital's experiences implementing a model program is described.

Medsurg Nurs 1997 Oct;6(5):256-67; quiz 268-9
Development of an ostomy competency.
Clayton HA, Boudreau L, Rodman R, Bak S, Embry K, Fortier J.
Northwestern Memorial Hospital, Chicago, IL, USA.
Staff educators and staff nurses developed an ostomy competency, with the guidance and expertise of the advanced practitioner and enterostomal nurse at a large teaching hospital. The competency improved the quality of care for surgical ostomy patients. Care was standardized and staff nurses' clinical knowledge was enhanced. Following the sessions, staff nurses verbalized increased confidence in working with patients with ostomies and demonstrated increased autonomy and problem-solving abilities. No variances in educational aspects of care were noted on clinical pathways.

Medsurg Nurs 1998 Feb;7(1):9-17; quiz 17-8
Breaking the boundaries: collaborating to develop a model ventilator training

program.
Roman M, Miller L, Macaluso S, Dempsey R, Golden-Baker S.
Massachusetts General Hospital, Boston, USA.
Changes in the health care system have created new opportunities for acute care nurses to establish collaborative relationships with their rehabilitation partners. When a rehabilitation facility decided to establish a ventilator weaning rehabilitation program, an acute care facility joined forces with the institution to develop an educational plan for the nursing staff. The development and implementation of the educational program as well as the collaborative relationship established between the two facilities are highlighted in this continuing education article.

Medsurg Nurs 2000 Jun;9(3):129-34
Surviving managed care: the effect on job satisfaction in hospital-based nursing.
Buiser M.
University of Pennsylvania, School of Nursing, Master's in Nursing and Health Care Administration Program, Philadelphia, USA.
Major changes brought about by managed care have redefined the nursing profession. Current trends such as case management, downsizing, restructuring of the workforce, and changes in the patient profile have had numerous effects, particularly on job satisfaction among hospital-based nurses. Strategies to improve job satisfaction during this era of increased managed care penetration include enhanced communication mechanisms, support from hospital administration, implementation of care models that promote professional nursing practice, adequate staffing, and competitive salaries and benefits.

N HC Perspect Community 1996 Mar-Apr;17(2):62-5
Preparing acute care nurses for community-based care.
O'Neill ES, Pennington EA.

N HC Perspect Community 1997 Jan-Feb;18(1):32-5

Nursing partnerships: education and practice.
Malloch K, Laeger E.
Maryvale Samaritan Medical Center, AZ, USA.

Ned Tijdschr Geneeskd 2000 Sep 9;144(37):1794-5
[Complementary therapies in the hospital:'if you can't beat them, join them'?]
[Article in Dutch]
van Dam FS.
Nederlands Kanker Instituut/Antoni van Leeuwenhoek ziekenhuis, afd. Psychosociaal Onderzoek en Epidemiologie, Amsterdam.
Some major cancer hospitals in the United States have established a department for complementary medicine as a service to their patients. Surveys in the Netherlands have shown that notably nursing staff and consumers consider the availability of complementary therapy in health care to be very important. Nevertheless, this appears to be an undesirable development as the effectiveness of these therapies has not been demonstrated and the therapists involved might interfere with regular patient therapy.

New Horiz 1997 Aug;5(3):281-6
Is nursing education adequate for pulmonary artery catheter utilization?
Ahrens TS.
Barnes-Jewish Hospital, Saint Louis, MO, USA.
OBJECTIVE: To review the literature addressing the nursing education of pulmonary artery catheterization.
DATA SOURCE: All pertinent English language articles dealing with nursing education and pulmonary artery catheterization were retrieved from 1983 through 1996.
STUDY SELECTION: Clinical studies related to nursing education in this field were selected. Only two studies addressing nursing knowledge of pulmonary artery catheterization have been published to date.
DATA EXTRACTION: Both studies suggest that an improvement in several

areas of nursing knowledge is necessary. Unfortunately, these studies are limited in scope and depth.

DATA SYNTHESIS: The adequacy of nursing education in hemodynamic monitoring, ranging from cognitive to technical issues, has not been addressed in a systematic fashion in the literature.

CONCLUSION: Nurses need a standardized hemodynamic monitoring curriculum. At present, education of nurses is primarily institutionally based. While national guidelines exist for hemodynamic monitoring, no mechanisms are in place to verify the skills of individual nurses. Since physicians depend on the knowledge and skill of the bedside nurse to obtain accurate information, any study evaluating the impact of pulmonary artery catheterization should first control for nursing knowledge. Since this information is not currently known, the precise impact of pulmonary artery catheterization cannot be assessed at this time.

NT Learn Curve 1999 Aug 4;3(6):10
Clinical governance. 4. Effective clinical practice--2.
Northcott N.

NT Learn Curve 1999 Nov 3;3(9):10
Clinical governance. 6. Effective staff--2.
Northcott N.

NT Learn Curve 1999 Nov 3;3(9):10
Clinical governance. 6. Effective staff--2.
Northcott N.

NT Learn Curve 1999 Oct 6;3(8):10
Clinical governance. 5. Effective staff--1.
Northcott N.

Nurs Adm Q 1997 Spring;21(3):29-49
LDS hospital, a facility of Intermountain Health Care, Salt Lake City, Utah.
Peck M, Nelson N, Buxton R, Bushnell J, Dahle M, Rosebrock B, Ashton CA.
Central Urban Regional Hospitals, Salt Lake City, Utah, USA.
On-line documentation by nurses and a comprehensive text management system are functional in several facilities of intermountain Health Care (IHC). The following articles detail factors in the design and implementation of this computerized network as experienced at LDS Hospital, part of the IHC system. Areas discussed are the system's applications for medical decision support, communication, patient classification, nurse staffing versus cost, emergency department usage, patient problem/event recording, clinical outcomes, and text publication. Users express satisfaction with the time saving, consistency of reporting, and cohesiveness of these applications.

Nurs Adm Q 1998 Summer;22(4):55-65
Improving clinical effectiveness through an evidence-based approach: meeting the challenge for nursing in the United Kingdom.
Gerrish K, Clayton J.
School of Health and Community Studies, Sheffield Hallam University, England.
Improving clinical effectiveness is a major challenge facing nurses working in the United Kingdom and requires a coordinated approach in order to ensure that the information about which interventions work is made available to those in a position to use it. This means that policy makers, administrators, and nurses need to base decision making on the best available evidence. In this article we explore the background to the drive for evidence-based practice and discuss how a group of nurse researchers have begun working with nurse administrators and practitioners in a large acute hospital to help change the rhetoric of evidence-based practice in nursing into reality.

Nurs BC 1999 Jan-Feb;31(1):16-9
Emergency nursing care of injection drug users: a positive approach.
McCall J.
Emergency Department, St. Paul's Hospital, Vancouver.

Nurs Case Manag 1997 May-Jun;2(3):122-6
Implementation of collaborative practice through interdisciplinary rounds on a general surgery service.
Felten S, Cady N, Metzler MH, Burton S.
University Hospital & Clinics, Columbia,

Missouri, USA.

Interdisciplinary teaching rounds were initiated on a general surgery service at a university teaching hospital. These rounds were designed to promote more efficient patient care by providing an opportunity for enhanced communication among health-care professionals. Improved collaboration is a prerequisite for implementation of critical paths and case management. The authors describe their methods of rounds development and the impact of the rounds on patient outcomes.

Nurs Case Manag 1999 Sep-Oct;4(5):236-41
Hospital-based nursing case management: role clarification.
Wayman C.
ccwayman@aol.com
Hospital-based nursing case management as a model of healthcare delivery has substantially grown over the last 10 years. Nursing case management as a viable professional role has developed along with this trend. In an era of decreasing reimbursements and increasing accreditation requirements, hospital administrators view nurse case managers as one answer to balancing cost and quality. However, the actual role and practice of nurse case managers within the hospital setting is inconsistent and often depends on the needs and expectations of the organization, as well as the level of experience and educational preparation of the nurse case manager.

Nurs Clin North Am 1996 Jun;31(2):387-403
Implementing a research-based kangaroo care program in the NICU.
Bell RP, McGrath JM.
Maricopa Medical Center, Phoenix, Arizona, USA.
Kangaroo care or skin-to-skin holding of preterm infants requires consistent implementation for best outcomes with infants and families. Successful implementation of a project of this type demands an organized approach. This article describes how a standard of care was developed using research findings and then implemented with a step-by-step approach in the neonatal intensive care

unit.

Nurs Clin North Am 1998 Mar;33(1):105-18
Effective peer responses to impaired nursing practice.
Smith LL, Taylor BB, Hughes TL.
Intervention Project for Nurses, Ponte Vedra Beach, Florida, USA.
Chemical dependency within the nursing profession continues to be a significant problem affecting health care delivery. This article presents up-to-date information on responding to a peer who is demonstrating impaired nursing practice. Specific information on the scope and impact of the problem, indicators of impairment, return to practice, and fitness to practice issues are addressed. In addition, the authors share their insight regarding progress, trends, and challenges in responding to impaired practice.

Nurs Clin North Am 1998 Mar;33(1):105-18
Effective peer responses to impaired nursing practice.
Smith LL, Taylor BB, Hughes TL.
Intervention Project for Nurses, Ponte Vedra Beach, Florida, USA.
Chemical dependency within the nursing profession continues to be a significant problem affecting health care delivery. This article presents up-to-date information on responding to a peer who is demonstrating impaired nursing practice. Specific information on the scope and impact of the problem, indicators of impairment, return to practice, and fitness to practice issues are addressed. In addition, the authors share their insight regarding progress, trends, and challenges in responding to impaired practice.

Nurs Clin North Am 1998 Mar;33(1):47-60
Substance abuse concerns in the treatment of pain.
Vourakis C.
Samuel Merritt College, Oakland, California, USA.
Current knowledge about the use of options for the management of patient pain opposes conventional practice, which is guided by misunderstandings and personal attitudes and beliefs. An understanding of

substance abuse and the behavior and needs of the person with substance dependence are important elements in a nurse's knowledge base. This understanding allows him/her to safely and effectively manage pain in all patients. Effective pain management education needs to be comprehensive and should include not only updated information, but also explore origins of beliefs about pain and substance abuse and how these beliefs affect current practice. This article discusses the common myths that often guide nurses' management of patient pain and offers strategies for care that are based on current understandings.

Nurs Crit Care 1996 Jan-Feb;1(1):26-30
Exploring the psychological effects of intensive care on paediatric patients: issues from the literature.
Palmer J.
Intensive Therapy Unit, Queen Alexandra Hospital, Portsmouth, Hampshire.
The psychological needs of children in intensive care may often be neglected in favour of a more physiological approach to nursing care. Both the short- and long-term psychological effects of paediatric intensive care require examination. There is a lack of research-based evidence on the psychological effects of intensive care on children. The intensive therapy unit (ITU) itself, developmental age, role of the family, loss of self-control/routine, under/over-use of sedation and analgesia, play, and the ITU nursing staff all have a significant psychological impact on the critically ill child. Strategies that reduce the negative psychological effects of ITU must address the above issues.
Publication Types: Review; Review Literature

Nurs Crit Care 1996 May-Jun;1(3):137-40
Death: a concept analysis and application to practice.
Gelling LH.
Transplant High Dependency Unit, Addenbrooke's Hospital, Cambridge.
Death is a commonly used concept but is surrounded by much mystery. The concept of death is examined using the Walker and Avant (1995) framework for concept analysis. The use of the concept death is considered in the intensive care unit. In the intensive care unit a conflict often exists between the curing culture and the inevitability of death.

Nurs Crit Care 1996 Nov-Dec;1(6):286-91
Brain stem death and organ donation.
Davies C.
Bristol Royal Infirmary.
Our understanding of the concept and definition of death has changed over time. The British contribution to the body of knowledge on the diagnosis of brain steam death was the publication by the medical royal colleges (1976) of diagnostic criteria. Most literature and research which explores the knowledge and attitudes of nurses towards the concept of brain stem death is from the USA. Several issues which arise from the literature are discussed in relation to organ donation. Further UK-based research is required.

Nurs Crit Care 1997 Jan-Feb;2(1):11-6
Nursing diagnosis: use and potential in critical care.
Mills C, Howie A, Mone F.
Intensive Care and Nursing Development Unit, Chelsea and Westminster Hospital, London.
Nursing diagnosis is a classification system for nursing widely used in the USA. There is increasing interest in its potential for use within British nursing. Benefits and concerns are raised about using nursing diagnosis in practice. This paper considers the potential for using nursing diagnosis in a critical care setting. Using nursing diagnosis raises many issues for British nurses, and these need to be discussed and clarified prior to implementation into practice.

Nurs Crit Care 1997 Jan-Feb;2(1):17-24
The physiological knowledge required by nurses caring for patients with unstable angina.
Todd N.
North Middlesex Hospital NHS Trust, London.
Physiological knowledge necessary to

critically analyse nursing management of patients with unstable angina is reviewed. The role of endothelium derived relaxing factor, nitrous oxide and atherosclerosis is summarised. The effects of circadian rhythms or clinical signs and symptoms in patients with unstable angina is particularly highlighted. Pharmacological interventions are considered from the perspective of implications for nursing care and other important nursing interventions identified for coronary care nurses.

Nurs Crit Care 1997 Jan-Feb;2(1):29-33
Nutritional assessment in clinical practice: a review.
Say J.
Department of Adult Nursing (South), University of Hertfordshire, Hatfield.
Malnutrition is a common problem within the clinical setting. Patients affected by malnutrition are more likely to suffer serious complications with an associated increase in length of stay and cost of treatment. Despite these serious outcomes, nurses are still failing to nutritionally assess their patients. This paper explores means of determining nutritional status in order to facilitate early detection and treatment of nutritional problems.

Nurs Crit Care 1997 Jan-Feb;2(1):34-7
Supervision in practice.
Pritchard T.
Intensive Care and Nursing Development Unit, Chelsea and Westminster Hospital, London.
The nature of the supervising relationship is explored in relation to an intensive care unit. The relationship between clinical supervision and individual performance review is discussed. Preparation and support for the supervisor's role is identified. Peer, group and external supervision arrangements are explored.

Nurs Crit Care 1997 May-Jun;2(3):112-9
The needs of parents with a child on an adult intensive therapy unit.
Plowright C.
Intensive Therapy Unit, Kent and Canterbury Hospital.
This review examines, by means of a literature search, the needs of parents who have a critically ill child on adult intensive therapy units. These needs are compared with the needs of relatives of adult patients in ITUs. Whether nurses trained in adult nursing have the necessary skills, knowledge and attitudes to care for the parents is also discussed. Recommendations for ensuring care of the parent point to addressing skills gaps in adult-trained nurses and to reappraising visiting policies.

Nurs Crit Care 1997 May-Jun;2(3):138-43; discussion 144-5
Reflections on being therapeutic and reflection.
Elcock K.
Wolfson School of Health Sciences, Thames Valley University, Ealing, London.
This article offers a reflective account of an incident that occurred between a nurse tutor and a patient on a cardiology ward. It highlights the importance of interpersonal skills in creating a therapeutic relationship, in particular those of self-awareness, empathy and intuition. The author's difficulties in running reflective practice sessions for pre-registration students are discussed and insights are offered into why these difficulties arose.

Nurs Crit Care 1997 May-Jun;2(3):146-9
Nurses' under-medication of analgesia in cardiac surgical patients: a personal exploration.
Cottle S.
St Thomas' Hospital, London.
This paper examines aspects of care which may account for some of the reasons why critical care nurses fail to relieve patients' pain following cardiothoracic surgery. Factors that may influence the critical care nurses' decision regarding the amount of opiate analgesia to give a patient are examined using the 'Theory of Planned Behaviour' as a framework for enquiry. The skills required by the critical care nurse in planning how to play the phenomena of 'the doctor-nurse game' may be a key element in meeting the goal of pain relief for the patient following cardiac

surgery.

Nurs Crit Care 1998 May-Jun;3(3):122-9
Addressing the sexual concerns of patients following myocardial infarction.
Ketchell A.
School of Health Care Studies, University of Leeds.
The review explores the dimension of sexuality for patients with a myocardial infarction. It discusses the role of the nurse in addressing issues of sexuality for this group. Potential reasons for the apparent difficulties faced by nurses and patients when dealing with this issue are considered. Tentative recommendations are made for closing the apparent gap between principles and practice.

Nurs Crit Care 1998 May-Jun;3(3):130-3
Intuition and the coronary care nurse.
Hams S.
Coronary Care Unit, Wiltshire Cardiac Centre, Princess Margaret Hospital, Swindon.
The paper sets out to explore the place of intuition in coronary care nursing. The Dreyfus (1985) and Benner (1984) models are used to explore the relevance of intuition to clinical practice. Examples from clinical practice are used to discuss the status of intuition in current practice. Conclusions suggest that further work is needed to explore the value of intuition and its contribution to clinical care.

Nurs Crit Care 2000 May-Jun;5(3):148-52
Addressing sexuality in intensive care: an addition to the curriculum.
McLuskey J, Viney C.
University of Nottingham, School of Nursing, Nottingham NG7 2UH.
A range of views of sexuality is explored, concluding that sexuality is more than sexual orientation. A review of the literature revealed that little attention is given by nurses in intensive care to meeting those needs of patients which relate to their sexuality. Vignettes, taken from practice, are given as examples of where the sexuality of a patient has been a significant element and these are used to examine nurses' attitudes to sexuality. An evaluation of two teaching sessions is given.

Nurs Econ 1991 May-Jun;9(3):175-8
Patient care automation: the future is now. Part 6. Does reality live up to the promise?
Korpman RA.
By almost any measure, it appears that patient-centered integrated information systems with an operations optimization focus contribute significantly to an institution's efficiency, efficacy, and quality. As with any other management enhancement tool, savings will only accrue if the institution manages to the savings. Nevertheless, such savings appear realizable and achievable. User communities, including nurses, physicians, administrators, and others all profit individually and collectively by using such a system. Finally, by providing better quality care and spending less time on clerical work, patients are the ultimate recipients of the benefits of an integrated patient-centered approach.

Nurs Econ 1997 Sep-Oct;15(5):253-61, 264
Differentiated nursing practice: assessing the state-of-the-science.
Baker CM, Lamm GM, Winter AR, Robbeloth VB, Ransom CA, Conly F, Carpenter KC, McCoy LE.
Indiana University School of Nursing, Indianapolis, USA.
The authors present their findings following an exhaustive literature review of research on differentiated nursing practice (DNP) that used a number of tools to measure various aspects of DNP that are applicable across the health care delivery continuum. Issues related to DNP include: optimal nursing care, matching patient needs with nurse competencies, effective use of nursing resources, equitable compensation, career satisfaction, loyalty to employers, and enhanced prestige of the nursing profession. One 1992 Massachusetts study of a three-role oncology unit project (including patient care manager, clinical nurse, and patient care technician), showed positive change in five criteria including: standards of nursing care, actual care hours, average labor costs,

job satisfaction and patient satisfaction. A 1990 Arizona study that included unit assistants concluded that DNP supported a decline in the use of supplemental staff and staff overtime which led to cost savings, and increases in the actual hours of care and nurse satisfaction.
Publication Types: Review; Review Literature

Nurs Econ 1998 Nov-Dec;16(6):291-7, 312
Policy implications when changing staff mix.
Hall LM.
Faculty of Nursing, University of Toronto, Ontario, Canada.
Publication Types: Review; Review Literature

Nurs Econ 1998 Sep-Oct;16(5):254-7, 253
The triad of empowerment: leadership, environment, and professional traits.
Fullam C, Lando AR, Johansen ML, Reyes A, Szaloczy DM.
Nurse Executive Program, Teachers' College/Columbia University, New York, NY, USA.
Empowerment is defined as "moving decision making down to the lowest level where competent decisions can be made." In the hospital setting, this would most commonly be at the point of direct patient care or staff nurse level; however, this kind of empowerment requires an environment of autonomy where mutual trust and respect are encouraged. The empowerment process requires that staff be prepared to accept and effectively use expanded decision-making responsibilities. The professional accountabilities of the empowered nurse include having a sense of value about their work and willingness to provide the full scope of practice as well as ability to work as equal members of a comprehensive interdisciplinary team. In order to move into a fully empowered position, professional nurses need mentoring, education, awareness of political activism opportunities, and networking skills.

Nurs Ethics 1996 Dec;3(4):285-93
Resolving the ethical dilemma of nurse managers over chemically-dependent colleagues.
Chiu W, Wilson D.
Faculty of Nursing, University of Alberta, Edmonton, Canada.
This paper addresses the nurse manager's role regarding chemically-dependent nurses in the workplace. The manager may intervene by: terminating the contract of the impaired colleague; notifying a disciplinary committee; consulting with a counselling committee; or referring the impaired nurse to an employee assistance programme. A dilemma may arise about which of these interventions is ethically the best. The ethical theories relevant to nursing involve ethical relativism, utilitarianism, Kantian ethics, Kohlberg's justice, and Gilligan's ethic of care. Nurse managers first need to understand these theories in order to clarify their own perceptions and attitudes towards chemical dependency, and then satisfactorily resolve this ethical dilemma. Education and social learning are routes to a better understanding of chemical dependency and to broadening the ethical dimensions of nurse managers.

Nurs Ethics 1998 Mar;5(2):95-102
The key to quality nursing care: towards a model of personal and professional development.
Glen S.
School of Nursing and Midwifery, University of Dundee, Ninewells, UK.
Quality of nursing cannot be assessed in terms of performance referenced criteria, but only in terms of the personal qualities displayed in the performance. The key to improvement in practice may be the improvement of emotional and motivational tendencies. In essence, professional development implies personal development. Harre makes a distinction between 'powers to do' and 'powers to be' (a state of being). The former are the capacities that individuals acquire to perform their tasks and roles. Professional development therefore involves, first, the acquisition of the capacities necessary for the successful completion of a set of professional tasks (the powers to do).

Secondly, it involves the acquisition of the appropriate emotions and motivations, and the theories about human nature and the conduct that underpins them (the powers to be). Therefore, these capacities cannot be derived from analysis of tasks, since what are defined as tasks in the first place are determined by the exercise of such powers. The acquisition of attitudes constitutes a source of competent practice. Harre's model of 'personal identity' provides a conceptual framework for thinking about the process of the acquisition of nursing competence and its relationship to differing views of nursing. Considerations relating to different priorities within Harre's model make it possible to raise questions about the objectives of competence at different stages.

Nurs Ethics 1999 Sep;6(5):374-82
Reflections on the meaning of care.
Sabatino CJ.
Daemen College, Amherst, New York 14226, USA.
Health care is increasingly delivered by using medical technologies and specialized procedures. However, the systems through which it is delivered are coming under attack as lacking in care. Medicine is very capable of treating the human body, but it may be losing its sensitivity towards persons, especially concerning the vulnerability they are experiencing. Nurses are finding that the demands for more efficiency and cost-effective measures do not allow them sufficient time to offer the personal care for which they have always felt responsible. The question of the meaning of care surfaces especially in treating those who are approaching death. The need is to balance the various dimensions of care, keeping its focus on the well-being of persons.

Nurs Inq 1999 Sep;6(3):167-77
Situating wound management: technoscience, dressings and 'other' skins.
Rudge T.
School of Nursing, Faculty of Health Science, Flinders University of South Australia, Australia.
Trudy.Rudge@flinders.edu.au

This paper addresses the notion of wound care as a technology of skin and other skins imbued with the combined power of technology and science. It presents the discourses of wound care evident in the accounts of patients and nurses concerning this care, and discussions about wounds in wound care interest groups, journals, and advertising material about wound care products. The discussion focuses on wounds and wound dressings as effects immanent in the power relations of discourses of wound care. These effects colour and influence nurses' responses to wounds and wound care products. Moreover, the discourses that portray these practices are evidence of the complex articulation between technoscience and gender. Nurses and patients are fascinated by wound technoscience and lured towards it by its potential for mastery and control over wounds. Such seductions are evident in the texts of nurses, patients, and pharmaceutical advertisements for wound care products. Finally, the ways that these representations are used to talk about and market wound care products are shown as exemplifying the finer points of wound management as a nursing technoscience.

Nurs Inq 1999 Sep;6(3):167-77
Situating wound management: technoscience, dressings and 'other' skins.
Rudge T.
School of Nursing, Faculty of Health Science, Flinders University of South Australia, Australia.
Trudy.Rudge@flinders.edu.au
This paper addresses the notion of wound care as a technology of skin and other skins imbued with the combined power of technology and science. It presents the discourses of wound care evident in the accounts of patients and nurses concerning this care, and discussions about wounds in wound care interest groups, journals, and advertising material about wound care products. The discussion focuses on wounds and wound dressings as effects immanent in the power relations of discourses of wound care. These effects colour and influence nurses' responses to wounds and wound care products.

Moreover, the discourses that portray these practices are evidence of the complex articulation between technoscience and gender. Nurses and patients are fascinated by wound technoscience and lured towards it by its potential for mastery and control over wounds. Such seductions are evident in the texts of nurses, patients, and pharmaceutical advertisements for wound care products. Finally, the ways that these representations are used to talk about and market wound care products are shown as exemplifying the finer points of wound management as a nursing technoscience.

Nurs Manag (Harrow) 1997 May;4(2):14-7
Towards evidence based practice.
Hunt J.
Nursing Research Initiative for Scotland, Glasgow.

Nurs Manag (Harrow) 1997 May;4(2):24-5
Leadership and team building.
Sheldon L, Parker P.
City University, St Bartholomew's School of Nursing.

Nurs Manag (Harrow) 1997 Sep;4(5):13-5
Clinical supervision for forensic mental health nurses.
Rogers P, Topping-Morris B.
Caswell Clinic, Bridgend & District NHS Trust.

Nurs Manag (Harrow) 1998 Jun;5(3):16-9
Implementing clinical effectiveness.
McClarey M.

Nurs Manag (Harrow) 1998 May;5(2):14-7
Education for the future.
Clark JM.
King's College London.
Publication Types: Lectures; Review
Review, Tutorial

Nurs Manag (Harrow) 1998 May;5(2):14-7
Education for the future.
Clark JM.
King's College London.
Publication Types: Lectures; Review
Review, Tutorial

Nurs Manag (Harrow) 1998 May;5(2):22-3
Providing effective clinical supervision.
Porter NJ.
University of Portsmouth School of Health Studies.

Nurs Manage 1997 Feb;28(2):45-9; quiz 50
Comment in: Nurs Manage. 1997 Sep;28(9):10
Does certification mean better performance?
Redd ML, Alexander JW.
Patient Care Services, Onslow Memorial Hospital, Jacksonville, North Carolina, USA.
This research addresses the efficacy of certification in nursing in terms of differences in job performance and self-esteem. Study results could help nurse managers determine hiring criteria, design professional development programs and restructure pay scales and reward systems.

Nurs Manage 1998 Apr;29(4):33-5; quiz 36
An equitable nursing assignment structure.
Davidhizar R, Dowd SB, Brownson K.
Bethel College, Mishawaka, Indiana, USA.
An inconsistent nursing assignment structure increases unsafe nursing care situations and patient and staff litigation. Using a holistic perspective when scheduling places value on subjectivity, accountability and continuity of care. The conflicts involved with the nursing assignment structure and its implications for nursing managers are identified.

Nurs Manage 1999 Feb;30(2):25-9; quiz 29-30
It's a match!
Howell SB.
Inpatient Services, Beebe Medical Center, Lewes, Del., USA.
When interviewing a candidate for employment, nurse managers must analyze a unit's strengths and weaknesses to find someone who not only fits the job description, but will be an asset to the unit.

Nurs N Z 1999 Jun;5(5):22-4
Workforce planning essential.
Peach J.
Waitemata Health.

Nurs Outlook 1995 Sep-Oct;43(5):201-9
Transformation of the nursing workforce.
Aiken LH.
Center for Health Services and Policy
Research, University of Pennsylvania,
Philadelphia, USA.
Publication Types: Review; Review
Literature

Nurs Outlook 2000 Jul-Aug;48(4):158-64
End-of-life decisions in adult intensive
care: current research base 158 and
directions for the future.
Baggs JG, Schmitt MH.
University of Rochester, School of
Nursing, Rochester, New York.
Publication Types: Review; Review,
Academic

Nurs Outlook 2000 Sep-Oct;48(5):199-201
Moral distress in everyday ethics.
Hamric AB.
University of Virginia School of Nursing,
Charlottesville, USA.

Nurs Outlook 2000 Sep-Oct;48(5):211-7
Retirement, the nursing workforce, and the
year 2005.
Minnick AF.
College of Nursing, Rush University,
Chicago, Illinois, USA.
This analysis of workforce projections
confirms that early employment
withdrawal by registered nurse baby
boomers could have a profound effect on
US health care. The available policy
mechanisms to encourage or discourage
any early withdrawal require several years
to implement, which makes timely
decisions imperative.

Nurs Outlook 2000 Sep-Oct;48(5):211-7
Retirement, the nursing workforce, and the
year 2005.
Minnick AF.
College of Nursing, Rush University,
Chicago, Illinois, USA.
This analysis of workforce projections
confirms that early employment
withdrawal by registered nurse baby
boomers could have a profound effect on
US health care. The available policy
mechanisms to encourage or discourage

any early withdrawal require several years
to implement, which makes timely
decisions imperative.

Nurs Spectr (Wash D C) 1998 May
18;8(10):12-4
Networking for career advancement.
Restifo V.

Nurs Spectr (Wash D C) 1999 Mar 22;9(6):12-
3; quiz 14
Partnership: making the most of mentoring.
Restifo V.
Association for Professionals in Infection
Control and Epidemiology in Washington,
DC, USA.

Nurs Stand 1997 Apr 9;11(29):46-8
Teaching practical skills: a guide for
preceptors.
Farley A, Hendry C.
School of Nursing and Midwifery,
University of Dundee, Ninewells Hospital.
Concern has been expressed that recently
qualified nurses may be deficient in
clinical skills. In this article the authors
explore psychomotor skills learning and
suggest strategies to support preceptors
who have responsibility for developing
such skills in students. The advice should
prove helpful to clinical staff who are
involved in teaching clinical skills to
nursing students.

Nurs Stand 1998 Apr 1-7;12(28):49-52, 54
Pressure sore incidence: a strategy for
reduction.
Arblaster G.
Trust Administration Centre, Walsgrave
Hospitals NHS Trust, Coventry.
In this article, the author discusses how the
Walsgrave Hospitals NHS Trust
implemented a strategy to reduce the
prevalence of hospital-acquired pressure
sores. The role of the tissue viability nurse
is emphasised as is the development of a
staff education programme.

Nurs Stand 1998 Aug 5-11;12(46):23-7
Food for thought.
Holmes S.
Canterbury Christ Church College.

Nurs Stand 1998 Feb 25-Mar 3;12(23):35-7
Blood pressure measurement: assessing
staff knowledge.
Gillespie A, Curzio J.
Nursing Services, Victoria Infirmary NHS
Trust, Glasgow.

Nurs Stand 1998 Jun 24-30;12(40):42-6
Clinical supervision: characteristics of a
good supervisor.
Sloan G.
In this review of the literature, the author
evaluates research into supervisor and
supervisee perceptions of the attributes of
good clinical supervisors. Nursing studies
are reviewed but, because of the relative
dearth of studies on the topic, the author
draws on the counselling, psychology and
psychotherapy literature to develop
comparisons.
Publication Types: Review; Review
Literature

Nurs Stand 1998 Mar 11-17;12(25):42-3
Radiotherapy nursing: understanding the
nurse's role.
Downing J.
Centre for Cancer and Palliative Care
Studies, Institute of Cancer Research,
London.
Radiotherapy nurses are integral members
of the multidisciplinary team. In this
article, the author describes the role and
makes recommendations for its future
development.

Nurs Stand 1998 Oct 28-Nov 3;13(6):50-3;
quiz 55-6
Training-needs analysis.
Pedder L.
Nurse Education Unit (Human Resources
Directorate), Taunton and Somerset NHS
Trust.
This article introduces training-needs
analysis (TNA) and places the process in
the broad context of a training strategy. It
aims to inform nurses on how the
principles of TNA can be applied to their
own practice.

Nurs Stand 1998 Sep 9-15;12(51):35-9; quiz
41-2
Handwashing.

Kerr J.
Lanarkshire Healthcare NHS Trust.
This article discusses the procedure and the
skills that are required to perform
handwashing effectively and outlines the
importance of this procedure in relation to
infection control. This article is the first of
three subjects relating to the principles and
practice of infection control.

Nurs Stand 1999 Apr 7-13;13(29):51-2, 55-6
Improving wound care through clinical
governance.
Newton H.
Royal Cornwall Hospital, Truro.
The fundamental role of nurse specialists is
to improve and maintain the quality of
patient care across the organisation.
Heather Newton looks at the specialist
nursing role in the light of the clinical
governance arrangements.

Nurs Stand 1999 Aug 18-24;13(48):43-5
Dealing with problems in clinical practice.
Lowry M.
Leeds Metropolitan University.
The identification of problems and how
they are dealt with is affected by the
individual perspectives of all parties
involved. Mike Lowry discusses how
groups of nurses often have difficulty
accepting that problems exist and suggests
ways they might go about identifying and
dealing with them.

Nurs Stand 1999 Feb 10-16;13(21):43-6
Violence at work.
Paterson B, McCornish AG, Bradley P.
In this article, the authors discuss violence
in healthcare settings and the health and
safety issues that are involved.

Nurs Stand 1999 Feb 10-16;13(21):49-54; quiz
55-6
Avoiding latex allergy.
Johnson G.
Occupational Health Services, University
Hospital, Aintree, Liverpool.

Nurs Stand 1999 Jul 14-20;13(43):48-53; quiz
54
Cardiopulmonary resuscitation: the
laryngeal mask airway.

Hand H.
School of Nursing and Midwifery,
University of Sheffield.

Nurs Stand 1999 Nov 17-23;14(9):42-4
Clinical supervision for professional
practice.
Jones A.
School of Nursing, Midwifery and Health
Visiting, University of Manchester.

Nurs Stand 2000 Mar 29-Apr 4;14(28 suppl):3-
17; quiz 18-25
We don't have to take this: dealing with
violence at work.
Brennan W.
Edenfield Centre, Salford Mental Health
Services.
The Health and Safety Executive has
identified nursing as the most hazardous
occupation in the United Kingdom. Nurses
are more likely to be on the receiving end
of violence than policemen (HSC 1997);
violence remains constant for employees in
healthcare. Most days there are news
reports of violent incidents being
perpetrated against nurses, doctors or other
NHS staff. If such incidents are not dealt
with adequately, the consequences can be
devastating, not only in terms of physical
injury to the victim, or psychological
trauma as a result of verbal abuse, but in
terms of morale and staff performance. As
they come face to face with violence,
nurses may feel increasingly isolated,
unsupported and uncared for. This
workbook aims to provide clear guidelines
for assessing the risk and dealing with the
hazard of violence for managers and
nurses. The menace of violence in
healthcare may never be eliminated
completely, but there are things that can be
done to manage, and therefore reduce the
problem.

Nurs Times 1991 Apr 24-30;87(17):67-8
Primary nursing. The steady advance of a
revolution.
Finch M.

Nurs Times 1996 Feb 14-20;92(7):34-5
Continuing education: how well is PREP
working?

Bagnall P, Garbett R.
It is nearly a year since the UKCC's
standards for post-registration education
were implemented. This paper reviews
some of the issues resulting from post-
registration education standards and
introduces a combined Nursing
Times/Queen's Nursing Institute study
looking at practitioner's access to
continuing education.

Nurs Times 1998 May 13-19;94(19):30-1
More nurses, more patients, more work.
Radcliffe M.

Nurs Times 1999 Dec 29-2000 Jan
5;95(50):55-7
Coaching for improving job performance
and satisfaction.
Girvin J.

Nurs Times 1999 Nov 17-23;95(46):54-5
Drugs administration: keeping pace with
change.
Evans A.
Wolfson Institute, Thames Valley
University.

Nurs Times 1999 Nov 17-23;95(46):54-5
Drugs administration: keeping pace with
change.
Evans A.
Wolfson Institute, Thames Valley
University.

Nurs Times 2000 Feb 3-9;96(5):47-50
NT opening learning: clinical supervision--
Part 2.
Glover D.

Nurs Times 2000 Mar 2-8;96(9):49-51
Roles and responsibilities.
Wolverson M.
Rotherham Priority Health Services NHS
Trust.

Nurse Educ Today 1998 Nov;18(8):655-62
Some thoughts on nurse-education/service
partnerships.
Cornes D.
Glasgow Caledonian University,
Department of Nursing and Community
Health, Glasgow, UK.

This paper discusses some of the issues involved in the design of the processes for developing effective partnerships between faculties of nursing and nursing provider organizations. After defining the term 'partnership' it considers, first, the advantages which can be realized from effective nurse-education/service partnerships. Secondly, it briefly explores how effective partnerships can be formed while suggesting that these prescriptions do not guarantee success. Finally, it argues that effective partnerships between nurse-education and service are most likely to be realized when their development is stated explicitly in the developmental strategy of the organizations involved.

Nurse Educ Today 1998 Oct;18(7):592-8
Keeping a reflective practice diary: a practical guide.
Heath H.
Homerton School of Health Studies (Cambridge), Education Centre, Addenbrooke's Hospital, UK.
Reflective practice aims to enhance client care via the professional development and growing expertise of practitioners. This paper offers practical guidelines for writing diaries that may form the basis for reflective practice, while acknowledging the skills that practitioners already use to examine their nursing actions and interactions. There is an emphasis on the outcomes of reflection as well as the reflections themselves, as this is seen as important if professional development is to be recognized and clients benefit. Time constraints that may make frequent formal reflection difficult are recognized by the format that allows deeper reflection where time permits and as skills develop. While ideas presented have been influenced by the literature on reflection, the paper owes as much to the continuing education students of the Homerton School of Health Studies who studied the reflective practice module during 1996. Without listening to their discussions, becoming aware of their difficulties and sharing their growing ability to reflect on practice, this article would not have been possible.

Nurse Pract Forum 1998 Dec;9(4):202-8
Nurse to acupuncturist: a personal transition.
Keuler H.
Jensen Health & Energy Center, Milwaukee, WI, USA.
Chinese medicine is an ancient medical system using acupuncture as one of its principal treatment modalities. Acupuncture is becoming increasingly popular in the United States as a treatment for pain and other physical problems. This article chronicles a professional transition from a hospital nursing career into that of Chinese medicine.

Nursing 2001 Feb;31(2):36-41; quiz 42
How to safeguard delivery of high-alert i.v. drugs.
Hadaway LC.
Hadaway & Associates, Milner, Ga., USA.

Nursingconnections 1997 Spring;10(1):5-12
A model of collaboration: the Academic Practice Council.
White BJ, Jarrett SL, Tolve CJ.
Department of Nursing, Regis University, Denver, CO, USA.
If the profession of nursing is to survive in the changing health care delivery system, new models of collaboration between nursing education and nursing practice must be developed. Nursing is both an academic discipline and a practice profession. The historic dissonance between education and practice has never served the profession of nursing; the pressing challenge is to blend one with the other now. In an effort to respond to the demands of the discipline and profession of nursing, an academic institution and a health care delivery system developed a model of interagency collaboration. This article addresses historical perspectives, and evolution, structure, activities, evaluation, and future plans to the Academic Practice Council.

Nursingconnections 1997 Spring;10(1):55-70
Collaborative partners in nursing education: a preceptorship model for BScN students.
LeGris J, Cote FH.

School of Nursing, McMaster University, Hamilton, Ont.

This article depicts and describes five significant steps in the process of establishing and maintaining a nursing student preceptor programme in a psychiatric unit. Specific collaborative relationships, roles, strategies, important qualities, and suggestions are identified to enhance the success and contributions of each of the three learning partners--student, preceptor, and clinical faculty tutor. The steps and processes highlighted in this model are based on the actual experience of a nurse educator in a university school of nursing, in collaboration with the director of psychiatry (also a nurse) at a community hospital in southern Ontario, Canada. The authors jointly share their perceptions of the strengths, limitations, and mutual benefits experienced throughout all phases of this collaborative partnership. In addition, student and preceptor feedback on the placement are described, demonstrating the usefulness of ongoing feedback from all the participants. This article will be of interest to other nurse educators planning to initiate and maintain clinical preceptorship programs.

Off J Can Assoc Crit Care Nurs 1998 Fall;9(3):24-8; quiz 29-30
The use of restraints in critical care.
Leith B.
A restraint is any physical or chemical measure used to limit activity or to control an individual's behaviour. Restraints may include locked rooms, locked chairs, mummy bags, jackets, vests, wristlets, anklets, belts, mitts, joint splints, or pharmacological agents. Clinical experience indicates that there is a high prevalence of restraint use in critical care areas. The use of restraints has become an important issue for health care professionals and is just beginning to be considered by critical care nurses. This article is intended to provide Canadian critical care nurses with a summary of the literature related to the use of restraints.

Off J Can Assoc Crit Care Nurs 1999 Spring;10(1):23-8

Do-not-resuscitate patients in critical care: moral and ethical considerations.
Mondor EE.
Royal Alexandra Hospital, Edmonton, Alberta.
In this article the author describes moral and ethical dilemmas presented by the "do-not-resuscitate" (DNR) patient in the critical care unit. The author defines the term DNR, and discovers implementation of the concept is not universally consistent among health care facilities. From the literature review, the author identifies characteristics, care requirements, economic cost, suitability of treatment, patient/family preferences, and health care professionals' values and beliefs as six important factors encompassing care and treatment of DNR patients in critical care. Recommendations for critical care professional practice, emphasizing the importance of communication, education, research, the development of specialized care units, and advance personal directives, is presented.

Off J Can Assoc Crit Care Nurs 1999 Summer;10(2):24-7
Challenging restricted visiting policies in critical care.
Chow SM.
University of Saskatchewan, Saskatoon.
The need for family members to visit their loved ones when they have been admitted into the critical care unit was identified in 1979 by Molter in the critical care family needs inventory (CCFNI). This need has been the centre of controversy for critical care units for many years. This article provides an overview of literature that refutes some of the rationales that have been used to restrict family visiting in the critical care unit. An overview of a liberalized (open, contract, inclusive or structured) visiting policy is discussed as an option to the restricted visiting policy.
Publication Types: Review; Review Literature

Ohio Nurses Rev 1998 Apr;73(4):3-6; quiz 11
Under oath: what a nurse witness must know.
Blackford M.

Autumn enterprises, Inc. North Canton, Ohio, USA.

Ohio Nurses Rev 1998 Jul;73(6):4-6; quiz 17-8
Nurses who become abusers: what can be done?
Harkulich J.

Ohio Nurses Rev 1999 Feb;74(2):4-5, 12-5; quiz 16
Erratum in: Ohio Nurses Rev 1999 May;74(5):2
Pain management--an overview.
Macklin EA.

Orthop Nurs 1996 Jan-Feb;15(1):23-8; quiz 29-30
Basic tools for the orthopaedic staff nurse.
Part I: Assertiveness.
Milstead JA.
Organizational restructuring and expanded settings of health care delivery provide opportunities for the orthopaedic staff nurse to review basic communication tools that are useful with clients and families, managers, and other health care providers. It is critical for the staff nurse to build a repertoire of skills that support leadership and encourage enlightened followers. This two-part article addresses assertiveness, conflict management, and negotiation skills that are basic to providing professional care with confidence and competence in a changing health care environment.

Orthop Nurs 1996 Jul-Aug;15(4):15-8
Same-day surgery: the nurse's role.
Dougherty J.
Outpatient surgery is one of the fastest growing trends In health care today. Providing preoperative and postoperative care to a diverse patient population in a limited amount of time presents numerous challenges. The nursing staff is required to assess the patient and resources, plan for the scheduled surgery and postdischarge care, implement the plan, and evaluate the patient's and family's understanding of the information and their ability to provide for self-care at home in as little as 2 hours. Preoperative care is discussed in this article along with specific guidelines for

postoperative recovery and discharge planning. Care of the orthopaedic patient is highlighted throughout the discussion.

Orthop Nurs 1996 Mar-Apr;15(2):39-45; quiz 46-7
Basic tools for the orthopaedic staff nurse-- Part II: conflict management and negotiation.
Milstead JA.
Duquesne University, Pittsburgh, Pennsylvania, USA.
Organizational restructuring and expanded settings of health care delivery provide opportunities for the orthopaedic staff nurse to review basic communication tools that are useful with clients and families, managers, and other health care providers. It is critical for the staff nurse to build a repertoire of skills that support leadership and enlightened followers. The second of this two-part article builds on "Part I: Assertiveness" and addresses conflict management and negotiation skills that are basic to providing professional care with confidence and competence in a changing health care environment.

Orthop Nurs 1998 Jul-Aug;17(4):22-6
Professional reflection: have you looked in the mirror lately?
Oermann MH.
College of Nursing, Wayne State University, Detroit, Michigan, USA.
To remain competent in practice, as the demands of that practice change, and to take advantage of new roles and opportunities in nursing, three behaviors are required on the part of the nurse: ability to evaluate one's own knowledge and skills for practice, an awareness of resources available for development of new competencies for practice, and a willingness to engage in this self-assessment. This article explores these behaviors essential for the professional development of the nurse and includes specific strategies for assessing one's own learning needs and meeting them.

Orthop Nurs 1998 Sep-Oct;17(5):38-51
Managing the human side of change.
Salmond SW.

Department of Nursing, Kean University, Union, New Jersey, USA.
Change initiatives (strategic plans) often fail, not because the idea was wrong, but because the change process failed to consider the human side of change. Achieving desired change outcomes requires an accentuation of transition management efforts or a focus on people. This article proposes 12 steps to managing transition and preparing "change-ready" employees and highlights strategies for both staff and managers to consider in the process.

Orthop Nurs 2000 May-Jun;19(3):73-8
Deep-vein thrombosis prevention in orthopaedic patients: affecting outcomes through interdisciplinary education.
Hohlt T.
Clarian Health Partners, Inc., Indianapolis, Indiana, USA. thohlt@clarian.com
Deep-vein thrombosis (DVT) is a serious problem that affects millions of people annually. Prophylaxis against DVT following major orthopaedic surgery can save lives and health care dollars. Proper application of the prophylactic regimen by nursing and the interdisciplinary team can be a major key in affecting the outcome of the orthopaedic patient. To obtain successful outcomes, the educational needs of each individual in the interdisciplinary team must be met. Also, being aware of each physician's practice patterns, implementing their individual preferences, and ensuring that all equipment is available and used in a consistent manner will enhance the desired outcome.

Ostomy Wound Manage 1998 Mar;44(3A Suppl):51S-58S
Beyond risk assessment: elements for pressure ulcer prevention.
McNees P, Braden B, Bergstrom N, Ovington L.
Applied Health Science, Seattle, WA 98104, USA.
Considerable emphasis has been placed on identifying individuals who are at risk for developing pressure ulcers. However, the generality of diagnostic discriminations and consequent intervention strategies may have resulted in less effective outcomes than otherwise would be possible. When such processes are carried out in a system devoid of the fundamental elements required for increased diagnostic/prescriptive precision and systematic improvement, practitioners are, at best, relegated to relying on external trial-based research to yield new "best practices." At worst, ineffective and costly practices continue without systematic evaluation and alteration. Several necessary elements of any empirically-based prevention system are addressed, and an attempt to integrate the elements into a system for field utilization is illustrated. If successful, the system will result in incremental improvements in the outcomes of prevention efforts over time.

Paediatr Nurs 1998 Dec-1999 Jan;10(10):30-3; quiz 34-5
Infection control.
Simpson C.
Queen's Medical Centre, Nottingham.

Paediatr Nurs 1999 Dec-2000 Jan;11(10):18-20
Nurses' attitudes to disability.
Holmes L.
Association of Spina Bifida and Hydrocephalus, London.
Publication Types: Review; Review Literature

Pathol Biol (Paris) 2000 Oct;48(8):721-4
[Nosocomial infections in cancerology]
[Article in French]
Vannetzel JM.
Clinique Hartmann, 26, boulevard Victor-Hugo, 92200 Neuilly-sur-Seine, France.
Although not specific, nosocomial infections are particularly common in patients with solid tumor. Chemotherapy-induced time periods of aplasia are usually of short duration and less important than those induced in patients with blood tumor. Recent changes regarding cancer therapy are determining factors in regard to nosocomial infections: patients are treated in day hospitals that must conform to the strictest prevention norms; most of the patients have an indwelling venous

catheter for months, which may therefore be at the origin of an infection. Prevention and education of the nursing staff within the context of a heavy workload must be a priority, requiring efforts from everyone in the medical team.

Pediatr Nurs 1998 Jan-Feb;24(1):96-9
Beyond hospital walls: educating pediatric nurses for the next millennium.
Herrman J, Saunders A, Selekman J.
Department of Nursing, University of Delaware, Newark, USA.
As pediatric units in acute care hospitals close, as lengths of stay shorten, and as increasing numbers of procedures are completed on an outpatient basis, faculty must find different learning experiences for their prelicensure students. Some programs have discontinued pediatric rotations, others are seeking clinical experiences in community settings. These community experiences hopefully produce a more well-rounded, globally thinking nurse to practice in the 21st century, yet they also raise a number of concerns.

Pediatr Nurs 1998 Jan-Feb;24(1):96-9
Beyond hospital walls: educating pediatric nurses for the next millennium.
Herrman J, Saunders A, Selekman J.
Department of Nursing, University of Delaware, Newark, USA.
As pediatric units in acute care hospitals close, as lengths of stay shorten, and as increasing numbers of procedures are completed on an outpatient basis, faculty must find different learning experiences for their prelicensure students. Some programs have discontinued pediatric rotations, others are seeking clinical experiences in community settings. These community experiences hopefully produce a more well-rounded, globally thinking nurse to practice in the 21st century, yet they also raise a number of concerns.

Postgrad Med J 1996 Apr;72(846):211-3
The specialist nurse in HIV/AIDS medicine.
Whitehead CM.
AIDS Clinical Group, Royal Liverpool University Hospital, UK.

The management of patients with human immunodeficiency virus infection requires a multidisciplinary holistic approach. Hospital-based specialist nurses can both co-ordinate and facilitate their hospital care, and also ensure early and effective discharge back into the community.

Postgrad Med J 1996 Jul;72(849):413-8
Telling relatives that a family member has died suddenly.
Marrow J.
Accident and Emergency Department, Arrowe Park Hospital, Merseyside, UK.
Persons dying suddenly are very likely to be taken to the nearest Accident and Emergency Department. The task of informing and counselling bereaved relatives therefore frequently falls to the staff of these Departments. Adequate preparation is important in allowing such situations to be dealt with in a sensitive and appropriate manner. Advice on coping with different aspects of sudden death is given and some common reactions discussed. Special problems are also considered (eg, the death of a child, criminal violence, communication difficulties). Aftercare must also not be forgotten and staff should receive training in the care of the bereaved.

Prof Nurse 1997 Jan;12(4):280-3
Using learning contracts in clinical practice.
Lowry M.
Leeds Metropolitan University.
A learning contract is focused on the process of learning as well as the content. Control is vested in the clinical learner. Learning contracts can be particularly useful for the newly qualified staff nurse.

Prof Nurse 1998 Dec;14(3):156-8
Meeting the needs of patients' relatives.
Greenwood J.
Cardiothoracic Unit, Castle Hill Hospital, Cottingham, Humberside.
Research into stress experienced by the relatives of patients in intensive care may be equally applicable to general wards. Patients are part of a family group and holistic care should include all family members. All nurses should review their

practice in relation to relatives' needs.
Publication Types: Review; Review
Literature

Prof Nurse 1999 Jun;14(9):618-21
Extubation in ICU: enhancing the nursing
role.
Cull C, Inwood H.
ITU, St John's Hospital, Livingston.
UKCC guidance gives a clear framework
within which nurses can enhance their
practice. Enhanced nurses can extubate
patients with appropriate training and
suitable protocols. Cost-effective, high-
quality care can be provided by nurses
working to the best of their professional
knowledge and skill.

Rech Soins Infirm 1998 Sep;(54):17-70
[The initial and continuing education of
hospital nursing personnel: alternating
practical work with education]
[Article in French]
Goudeaux A.
Ecole des Cadres de Sante de la
Salpetriere, Paris.
Who, as a trainer, has never heard this
irritating leitmotiv on the lips of those who
work in the area? Therefore, each of them
is convinced that the other is wrong or does
not do what he should. Beyond the
anecdote, the problem of the difficult
conjunction between school and the real
world is posed. Two places and two logics:
the first one is concerned with learning, the
second one considers production as its
daily objective. But the words of our
imaginary interlocutor also remind us of
the confrontation between two fields:
theory and practice and their apparently
irrecondilable nature. Two disconnected
worlds in which the students come and go
with the frequent impression that they live
two lives. There is a lot of professional
literature on the subject of the "hands on"
theory of education. The pedagogical
device to which we refer enables the
trainee to eventually make a link between
what he learns at school and what he does
during his training period. Once this has
been asserted, it seems to us that the
problem still remains unresolved. How can
you create links between theory and

practice? Which skills are required for the
trainers? Which training device is
necessary? The hypothesis of the paper we
are presenting is that the question of work
is at the centre of the problematics of
"hands on" education. Work appears as the
interface between the world of school and
the one of field work. This assertion means
that the practive produces knowledge just
as research does and we must therefore
accept that the practitioners carry on their
work thanks to the accumulation, the
construction and the transmission of this
practical knowledge. Assuming that the
question of work serves as a link between
theory and practive means reconciling the
vision of the teacher and the one of the
practitioner. It implies that the trainer must
make the effort of going on the field to
observe, to understand and formalize what
this knowledge coming from the daily
experience is made of. This know-how is
the result of the mobilization of the
intelligence of the operators who are faced
all the time with the hazards of real life. In
the following work, we intend to put a
pedagogical practice to the test of reality,
according to the above mentioned
hypothesis, to test its effectivity, to sort out
the possibilities of change it enables it
imposes and to mark its limits. Our wish is
not to make the absolute proof of the
validity of a point of view. We know by
experience that the reality often escapes its
observer and that trying to get in contact
with it to possibly change it, means that
you must be faced with it through action,
and you must admit that success will not
always be the result of your attempts.

Rev Enferm 1999 Feb;22(2):91-7
[Organizational culture and professional
development in nursing]
[Article in Spanish]
Ruiz Moreno J.
Servicio de Medicina Intensiva, Hospital
Sagrado Corazon, Barcelona.
There is a lot of talk about the importance
of persons in organization and leadership,
nothing that the keys to lead the
organizational milieu in a positive and
beneficial manner have been established
for several decades. These keys are related

to the values of nursing as a profession and to how these may constitute intangible assets. Nonetheless, identifying such values and intangible assets is not the exclusive responsibility of business managers in the nursing field.

Rev Enferm 1999 Jan;22(1):11-5
[Organizational culture and professional development in nursing]
[Article in Spanish]
Ruiz Moreno J.
Servicio de Medicina Intensiva, Hospital Sagrado Corazon, Barcelona.

Rev Enferm 1999 Mar;22(3):170-4
[Organizational culture and the professional development in nursing]
[Article in Spanish]
Ruiz Moreno J.
Servicio de Medicina Intensiva, Hospital Sagrado Corazon, Barcelona.
In previous articles in (ROL 22(1)-22(2)) reference was made to the importance of the organizational milieu as a business policy, particularly in the nursing field. The values of nursing professionals were also mentioned, as well as how to establish these as intangible assets. Although not exclusively, the responsibility to identify these values lies in the hands of nursing administrators. The purpose of identifying the intangible assets of nursing is that these become a useful tool to change or guide the organizational setting in order to better execute the mission of health organizations in a more favorable way. This mission must be related to offering the best possible care and treatment to the community which is being served.

Rev Esc Enferm USP 1998 Apr;32(1):84-90
[Ergonomics and the occupational activities of the nursing staff]
[Article in Portuguese]
Alexandre NM.
This paper discusses some of the ergonomics conditions that contribute to the development of musculoskeletal disorders of the vertebral column and relates these conditions to the occupational activities of the nursing staff.

Rev Lat Am Enfermagem 1998 Jan;6(1):91-7
[Accumulation of data about adolescence by nurses: period from 1983 to 1996]
[Article in Portuguese]
Cano MA, Ferriani M das G, Alves AC, Nakata CY.
Departamento de Enfermagem Materno-Infantil e Saude Publica da Escola de Enfermagem de Ribeirao Preto da Universidade de Sao Paulo.
In the last ten years adolescence has been object of study of many researchers and considered by National and International Organizations as an age band with priority to actions of promotion, prevention and protection. Many factors contributed to this concern with adolescence, between them, we can emphasize the importance of this populational contingent that represents 30% of world population, besides the questions of precocious pregnancy, AIDS and drugs. As nurse researchers, we are interested in experiencing and characterizing quantitatively and qualitatively the scientific production about adolescence in nursing, using as source of data collection the national specific nursing periodicals. Data obtained in this research show that the adolescence theme is not explored by the nursing staff, and the most important aspects are related to sexuality.

Rev Lat Am Enfermagem 1998 Jan;6(1):91-7
[Accumulation of data about adolescence by nurses: period from 1983 to 1996]
[Article in Portuguese]
Cano MA, Ferriani M das G, Alves AC, Nakata CY.
Departamento de Enfermagem Materno-Infantil e Saude Publica da Escola de Enfermagem de Ribeirao Preto da Universidade de Sao Paulo.
In the last ten years adolescence has been object of study of many researchers and considered by National and International Organizations as an age band with priority to actions of promotion, prevention and protection. Many factors contributed to this concern with adolescence, between them, we can emphasize the importance of this populational contingent that represents 30% of world population, besides the questions of precocious pregnancy, AIDS

and drugs. As nurse researchers, we are interested in experiencing and characterizing quantitatively and qualitatively the scientific production about adolescence in nursing, using as source of data collection the national specific nursing periodicals. Data obtained in this research show that the adolescence theme is not explored by the nursing staff, and the most important aspects are related to sexuality.

RN 1998 Jul;61(7):21-4
Ethics in action. You overhear two nursing colleagues speaking disrespectfully about a grossly obese patient.
Haddad A.
School of Pharmacy and Allied Health Professions, Creighton University, Omaha, USA.

RN 2001 Feb;64(2):58-63; quiz 64
Impaired nurses: reclaiming careers.
Sloan A, Vernarec E.

SCI Nurs 1996 Dec;13(4):101-4
Paradigm for SCI nurse competency on adult-geriatric SCI rehabilitation unit.
Thomason SS, Binard JE, Gregg B, Padios E, Trotman J.
James A Haley Veterans Hospital in Tampa, Florida, USA.
This article is based upon an SCI Model Project, funded by the American Association of Spinal Cord Injury Nurses (AASCIN). The purpose of this project was to develop a model to validate theoretical and practical knowledge of Registered Nurses and Licensed Practical Nurses/Licensed Vocational Nurses in an SCI rehabilitation setting. The investigators were direct care providers in a 68 bed SCI rehabilitation service at the James A. Haley Veterans Hospital in Tampa, Florida. The theoretical framework was based upon three aspects: Competency Validation, Theoretical Knowledge, and Practical Knowledge. Competency Validation was directed towards incorporating the elements of assessment, maintenance, demonstration, and improvement of competencies on an ongoing basis. Theoretical knowledge encompassed the cognitive and

psychomotor aspects of SCI nursing, and Practical Knowledge highlighted the application of principles of caregiving. Two instruments were developed to harmonize theoretical and practical dimensions for competency validation: SCI Knowledge/Skill Appraisal (SKA) and Expertise in SCI Nursing Practice (ESNP). The purpose of this project was to design a model for validating theoretical and practical knowledge of Registered Nurses (RN's) and Licensed Practical Nurses/Licensed Vocational Nurses (LPN/LVN's) in an SCI rehabilitation setting. The investigators were direct care Licensed Practical Nurses/Licensed Vocational Nurses (LPN/LVN's) in an SCI rehabilitation setting. The investigators were direct care providers in a 68 bed spinal cord injury (SCI) rehabilitation service at the James A. Haley Veterans Hospital in Tampa, Florida.

SCI Nurs 1997 Mar;14(1):3-7
Development and implementation of nursing consultation groups on a spinal cord injury unit.
Govoni AL.
Stress, time constraints, patient satisfaction, need for support, and cost containment became the impetus for a nursing consultation group on a spinal cord injury (SCI) unit. This unit is located in part of a center for rehabilitation in a large, tertiary care medical center. Staff on this unit care for a maximum of 20 spinal cord injured individuals and their families. This article describes how the clinical nurse specialist (CNS) identified the need for such a group as well as the benefits, membership, structure, and types of nursing issues addressed. Pitfalls and how to avoid them are identified for those interested in developing similar consultation groups.

Semin Nurse Manag 1997 Mar;5(1):18-24
Managing communication in times of rapid change.
Keeling EB, Linnen B.
Keeling Consulting Group, Hewitt, TX 76643-3723, USA.
Change is typically perceived as frontline

staff learning and using new skills. The reality is that it means that managers must change first. The rapid and multidimensional changes that are occurring in health care today are affecting the way managers need to manage communications with their staff. It is no longer possible to manage communications between you and your staff in the same way. Managers need to attend to the emotional reactions and the concerns of people that are engendered by the changes. The ability to lead staff forward in the change, by managing communications, will be an indicator of managerial effectiveness and success.

Semin Nurse Manag 1999 Dec;7(4):179-82
The role of nursing administrators in empowering scholarly productivity among clinicians.
Davidhizar RE, Bechtel GA, Lillis PP.
Division of Nursing, Bethel College, Mishawaka, IN, USA.
The authors discuss strategies nursing administrators can use to promote scholarly productivity among their nursing staff. By incorporating mentoring, promoting collegial teams, involving nurses in the development of goals for scholarly activity, promoting professionalism, and modifying assignments to ensure time for research and writing, nurse executives can significantly enhance scholarly productivity in their professional nursing staff.

Semin Nurse Manag 1999 Jun;7(2):59-62
The 'super nurse' syndrome.
Davidhizar R, Shearer R.
Bethel College, Mishawaka, IN 46545-5591, USA.
The authors describe the dynamics of the "super nurse" syndrome and provide nurse managers experiencing this syndrome with strategies to assist them. The article discusses the roles of nurse educators, hospital development staff, mentors, and social support networks. The authors hope to prevent the "super nurse" syndrome from affecting new graduates, through proper education of nurse educators,

mentors, and nurse managers who assist the new graduates in problem solving and adjusting to being a "real nurse."

Semin Nurse Manag 1999 Jun;7(2):78-80
Change and professional development: an adult education approach.
Dowd SB.
Division of Medical Imaging and Therapy, University of Alabama, Birmingham 35294-1270, USA.
The purpose of this article is to explain the staff development approach as a means of enhancing the nurse manager's professional growth as well as the growth of employees. Staff development is growth-oriented, provides opportunity for self-direction, and integrates the needs of the learner and the facility while focusing on long-term goals. The author discusses integrating the goals of the adult learner and those of the health care organization as a means of meeting the needs of the institution and the individual employee.

Semin Nurse Manag 1999 Jun;7(2):81-5
When the nurse manager must help staff cope with change.
Davidhizar R, Shearer R, Dowd SB.
Bethel College, Mishawaka, IN 46545-5591, USA.
The authors describe the dynamics of change, barriers and resistance to change, and provide techniques for assisting staff cope with change. The nurse manager should provide support during change, intervene when change is a surprise, help staff find challenge in change, encourage staff to have courage and stamina while coping with change, and foster teamwork. Using these techniques enables the manager and staff to view change as a challenge and an opportunity rather than a threat.

Semin Oncol Nurs 1996 Aug;12(3):193-201
Home infusion therapy.
Gorski LA, Grothman L.
Covenant Home Health Care, Milwaukee, WI, USA.
OBJECTIVES: To examine issues related to the planning of an effective home infusion therapy program and to provide an

overview of specific home infusion therapies for patients with cancer. DATA SOURCES: Published articles, research studies, guidelines, and standards pertaining to infusion therapies. CONCLUSIONS: Advances in technology have expanded and increased the scope and success of home infusion therapy. Antimicrobial therapy, chemotherapy, pain management, total parenteral nutrition, and blood transfusion therapy are commonly administered to cancer patients at home. IMPLICATIONS FOR NURSING PRACTICE: A competent and experienced nursing staff is the cornerstone of a successful home infusion program. Safe provision of infusion therapy and care can be assured through selection of appropriate patients, effective patient education, well-defined agency policies, and effective coordination of home care services.

Semin Perioper Nurs 1996 Apr;5(2):98-101
Cadaver organ donation and moral distress: a staff nurse's perspective.
Boswell S.
Current advancements in medical science, such as the progress seen in the area of organ transplantation, brings with it many ethical dilemmas for which there are no precedents. Obtaining informed consent for cadaver organ donation requires perioperative nurses to confront the moral responsibility that they have to their patients, their patients' families, and to the nursing profession as a whole. The perioperative nurse must question his or her own moral and cultural beliefs, face their own fears of death, and confront societal misconceptions about brain death. This evolution is emotionally demanding and often stresses one's support systems. However, with self-discovery and education, it can also be very rewarding.

Semin Perioper Nurs 1996 Jul;5(3):152-6
Job satisfaction: a possibility?
Johnston CL.
Registered nurse job satisfaction is one of the most written about topics in the nursing literature. Is it possible to achieve in an organizational setting? Can the administrative structures control this phenomenon? This article suggests that job satisfaction is strongly influenced by individual perceptions of certain key variables. In addition, job satisfaction is presented as a responsibility of each individual nurse.

Semin Perioper Nurs 1996 Oct;5(4):218-21
Perioperative nursing--the Jamaican perspective.
Lopez SA.
Department of Advanced Nursing, University of the West Indies, Mona, Jamaica.
Under constraints of a restricted economy Jamaica strives to deliver health care at the standard of developed countries. Nurses in Jamaica assume various roles as they provide perioperative nursing care; they work as a team and act as patient advocates. Bonds of caring and love are often established between patients, families, and the nursing staff. The quality of nursing care often determines the client's perioperative outcome, and Jamaican nurses strive to meet the challenges inherent in achieving positive patient outcomes.

Semin Perioper Nurs 1997 Apr;6(2):102-4
Computers in the operating room: the staff nurse perspective.
Jones SE.
Surgery Flight, Vandenberg AFB, CA, USA.
Computers and information management are long-standing tools for the Perioperative Manager. As paperless nursing documentation makes its way into the operating room, the staff nurse must become adept at the use of the computer. How to get the staff nurse comfortable with this new role, and concerns the staff nurse may voice are the subject of this article.

Semin Perioper Nurs 1998 Oct;7(4):239-53
Are nurses knowledgeable in regards to latex allergy?
Lewis LC, Norgan G, Reilly M.
Nursing Service, Audie Murphy Division, South Texas Veterans Health Care System, San Antonio 78284, USA.

Lack of knowledge concerning latex allergy may lead to a life-threatening adverse reaction to natural rubber latex. Registered nurses need a latex allergy knowledge base to provide latex-safe health care to clients and to create a latex-safe environment. This research explored the current knowledge base of registered nurses as related to (1) the care of clients at risk for latex allergy, or diagnosed with latex allergy, and (2) the provision of a latex-safe environment for all populations. This article describes this research and its implications for nurses. A copy of the Latex Allergy Knowledge Base Self-Assessment Questionnaire is included at the conclusion of the article.

Semin Perioper Nurs 1999 Apr;8(2):71-9
Keeping them in stitches: humor in perioperative education.
Beitz JM.
Graduate Program, School of Nursing, La Salle University, Philadelphia, PA, USA.
Humor is one of the most effective teaching strategies available to perioperative nurse educators. Humor can be used to teach nursing students, surgical staff, and patients. This article describes the incorporation of humor into perioperative education and presents examples of specific humorous teaching strategies.

Semin Perioper Nurs 1999 Oct;8(4):183-92
Reading and understanding blueprints.
Madrid EM, Harkey L.
Burlington Medical Center, IA 52601, USA.
There is a common body of knowledge that must be familiar to all when interpreting architectural plans. Although health care practitioners may be experts in their own field, they may be unfamiliar with facility planning and design and therefore lack understanding of how to communicate effectively with the architectural team. The information provided is intended to familiarize nurses and other health care professionals with basic terminology and to provide an understanding of how to identify areas, structures, and dimensions on architectural plans.

Semin Perioper Nurs 2000 Jan;9(1):27-36
Malignant hyperthermia: a case study.
Martin SN, Vane EA.
Army Nurse Corps, Colorado Springs, CO, USA.
Malignant hyperthermia continues to be a life-threatening emergency that can occur without warning. With early discharge, this crisis may even occur at home. Perioperative, anesthesia, and Post-Anesthesia Care Unit (PACU) nursing staff need to be educated in the signs, symptoms, treatment, and care of a malignant hyperthermia patient. This is a US government work. There are no restrictions on its use.

Servir 1996 May-Jun;44(3):148-54
[From beginner to expert]
[Article in Portuguese]
Benner P.

Soc Sci Med 1999 Feb;48(3):363-74
Complaints against nurses: a reflection of 'the new managerialism' and consumerism in health care?
Beardwood B, Walters V, Eyles J, French S.
Division of Social Science, York University, Toronto, Ontario, Canada.
bbeardw@yorku.ca
This paper discusses the effects of restructuring on nursing as a profession through an examination of the issue of complaints in Ontario. It argues that new managerialist techniques and associated changes in the nature of work are reducing the autonomy of nurses and making it difficult for them to meet the standards of their profession. Simultaneously, the Ontario government has increased the power of the public in the disciplinary process and the College of Nurses of Ontario is encouraging patients to register their complaints. The growth of consumerism in health care, coupled with the disciplinary process, individualizes complaints and deemphasizes their relationship to restructuring. Moreover, in response to the increasing number of complaints - complaints which more often

come from the public - nursing organizations have encouraged the legalization of the disciplinary process, thus fostering the individualization of the issues.

Subst Use Misuse 2000 Mar;35(4):503-32
Nurses' attitudes toward substance misusers. II. Experiments and studies comparing nurses to other groups.
Howard MO, Chung SS.
George Warren Brown School of Social Work, Washington University, St. Louis, Missouri 63130, USA.
howard@gwbmail.wustl.edu
Experimental investigations of nurses consistently indicate that a patent labeled as a substance misuser is perceived far more negatively across a range of personal attributes than an identical patient who is not so labeled. Comparative evaluations suggest that nurses are less tolerant of social drinking and drug use and are more morally condemnatory of the chemically dependent than are other health-care professionals.

Urol Nurs 1998 Dec;18(4):291-5
The culture of long-term care: impact on a continence care program.
Smith DB.
DesChutes Medical, Bend, OR, USA.
Continence care in long-term care settings is a major caregiver and economic burden, with incontinence affecting an estimated 50% to 70% of all residents. Traditionally the continence care of residents is assigned to the nursing assistants and continence programs have been on paper only. These programs have had dismal success rates. Factoring in the culture of the long-term care setting can make the continence program more comprehensive and improve success rates.

AUTHOR INDEX

TITLE INDEX

A

A challenge for clinical nurses: a new nursing role, 49

A controlled evaluation of a lifts and transfer educational program for nurses, 48

A down-to-earth approach to being a nurse educator, 18

A enfermagem como profis: são (estudo num hospital-escola), 8

A Financial guide for nurses: investing in yourself and others, 1

A model for teaching critical thinking in the clinical setting, 45

A model of collaboration: the Academic Practice Council, 99

A practical guide to venepuncture and management of complications, 33

A review of intensive care nurse staffing practices overseas: what lessons for Australia?, 29

A review of preceptorship in undergraduate nursing education: implications for staff development, 68

A train of events?, 36

Accepting the challenges of pain management, 30

Action research applied to a preceptorship program, 75

Action research from the inside: issues and challenges in doing action research in your own hospital, 62

Acute symptom assessment: determining the seriousness of the presentation, 85

Addressing sexuality in intensive care: an addition to the curriculum, 92

Addressing the sexual concerns of patients following myocardial infarction, 92

Administration, 9, 71, 87, 96

Advance, the nurse's guide to success in today's job market, 12

Advancing your career: concepts of professional nursing, 10

An equitable nursing assignment structure, 95

Anatomy of a job search: a nurse's guide to finding and landing the job you want, 2

Application of pulse oximetry and the oxyhemoglobin dissociation curve in respiratory management, 44

Are nurses knowledgeable in regards to latex allergy?, 108

Aspects of pulmonary artery catheterization in critical care, 53

Assessing competence. Meeting the unique needs of nurses in small rural hospitals, 30

Assisting demented patients with feeding: problems in a ward environment. A review of the literature, 60

Australian nurses and device use: the ideal and the real in clinical practice, 28, 29

Avoiding latex allergy, 97

Awareness: the heart of cultural competence, 21

B

Back to the future: a framework for estimating health-care human resource requirements, 38

Backstage in the theatre, 61

Basic tools for the orthopaedic staff nurse. Part I: Assertiveness, 101

Basic tools for the orthopaedic staff nurse--Part II: conflict management and negotiation, 101

Becoming an A & E nurse, 23

Being the boss is not what it used to be!, 80

Beyond hospital walls: educating pediatric nurses for the next millennium, 103

Beyond risk assessment: elements for pressure ulcer prevention, 102

Bibliography on occupational health nursing, 13

E

F

O

P

U

V

W

Y

SUBJECT INDEX

A

administration, 8, 71, 87, 96

B

bibliography, 1, 2, 4, 8, 9, 11-13, 15-20

C

career changes, 1, 8
career choice, 6, 9, 11, 14, 19
career development, 6, 10
career mobility, 3, 8-10, 13, 16, 19
case management, 14
clinical competence, 6

D

Delivery of Health Care, 19

E

economics, nursing, 14
education, nursing, 4-6, 11, 12, 14, 15, 19
education, nursing, continuing, 6
employment, 14, 17, 19
entrepreneurship, 8
essays, 5

F

faculty, 14, 18
faculty, nursing, 14, 18

G

Great Britain, 6

H

health care teams, 11
health planning, 19
history, 6
hospitals, 12, 36, 47, 88, 96

I

industrial nursing, 13
infection control, 102
interprofessional relations, 16

J

job Application, 2
job hunting, 2, 8, 12
job satisfaction, 3, 9, 71, 108

L

leadership and team building., 95

M

Managed Care Programs, 14
methods, 28, 34, 42, 46, 52, 53, 57, 61, 68, 70, 78, 82, 84, 89

N

new business enterprises, 8
nurse and nursing, 2, 3, 14
nurse Clinicians, 13
nurse practitioners, 14
nurse, 2, 3-5, 10, 14, 27, 31, 36, 39, 41-43, 45, 55, 59, 60, 62, 63, 66-68, 70, 74, 77-79, 88, 89, 91, 94, 95, 98, 100-102, 106, 108-110
nursing audit, 15